THE
PRAM
DIET

THE
PRAM
DIET

REBECCA MUGRIDGE

BANTAM
SYDNEY AUCKLAND TORONTO NEW YORK LONDON

A Bantam book
Published by Random House Australia Pty Ltd
Level 3, 100 Pacific Highway, North Sydney NSW 2060
www.randomhouse.com.au

First published by Bantam in 2009

Addresses for companies within the Random House Group can be found at www.randomhouse.com.au/offices

National Library of Australia
Cataloguing-in-Publication Entry

Mugridge, Rebecca, 1980–.
The pram diet.

ISBN 978 1 86325 687 2 (pbk).

Mothers – Health and hygiene.
Exercise for women.
Diet.
Self-help techniques.

613.7045

Cover photograph by Kiren Chang
Cover design by Christabella Designs
Internal design by Midland Typesetters, Australia
Typeset in 11/15 pt ITC Garamond by Midland Typesetters, Australia
Printed and bound by Griffin Press, South Australia

Random House Australia uses papers that are natural, renewable and recyclable products and made from wood grown in sustainable forests. The logging and manufacturing processes are expected to conform to the environmental regulations of the country of origin.

10 9 8 7 6 5 4 3 2 1

Note to readers
The information contained in this book is not intended as a substitute for consulting with your healthcare provider, and is based on the author's own experiences. Always check with your healthcare provider before embarking on major dietary changes or exercise regimes, and seek professional help if you experience prolonged symptoms that you think might be depression. While care has been taken to provide accurate and safe information, the author, copyright holder and publisher do not accept responsibility for any problems arising out of the contents of this book.

For my daughter, Lily

I didn't know that your tears would hurt more than my own. I didn't know my favourite sound would be your laughter. I didn't know I would be forever wanting to check you while you slept, nor that I would feel a little lost whenever we are apart. I didn't know that my heart could hold so much love. That the world would freeze around me if I saw you fall. I didn't know I'd look back on my life before you, and wonder how it ever felt full.

But I do know I love you completely, and I always will.

Contents

Introduction

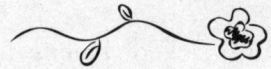

The breathtaking bond that consumes a woman as she holds her newborn baby is simply beautiful. Feelings of joy, hope and awe race through her body, igniting adrenaline-fuelled surges of emotion that seem to create a timeless bubble of bliss.

For me, the first two precious months of motherhood became a blur of the purest and deepest happiness I have ever known. Holding my daughter asleep in my arms, I felt complete peace. My partner Damien and I were happier than we had ever been.

But the realisation that this tiny person depends on you, and will learn from you the values and life skills needed to successfully guide them to adulthood, brings with it a great feeling of responsibility.

As a new mother, I became painfully aware that my lifestyle was not an ideal model for a healthy, active and happy life.

By the time Lily was a couple of months old, stress, exhaustion and fatigue had combined with diminishing self esteem and feelings of unattractiveness and sluggishness to leave me feeling depressed. There was an overall sense of heaviness I could not seem to lift. Slowly but surely, this downward spiral began to affect my ability to truly enjoy the blessings of my new child.

One day, utterly sick of feeling frustrated, angry and depressed, I put Lily in the pram, packed it up with spare bottles, blankets, nappies, dummies, teddies, water, sunscreen, a blanket, toys – even a first aid kit – and we went for our first big walk together. This walk wasn't a means to an end or a method of transportation – it was just a walk for walking's sake. It wasn't a marathon, but it was a big walk for us. I couldn't believe how amazing it felt, walking in that glorious fresh air, looking at the graceful, mighty trees, gazing at the endless horizon, hearing the wondrous sounds of nature all around us, smelling the wild, fresh scents, feeling the sun on my skin and the breeze in my hair. I could literally feel layers of stress and ill feelings peeling off me.

I had found a way to change my life for the better. A way to lift the dark feelings that had been draped around me and raise myself up to a new place where I was vibrant, healthy and, best of all, felt like a beautiful woman who was truly enjoying being a mother to my precious little daughter. I felt proud to be me and knew with confidence that I could and would, after all, be the great role model I wanted to be for my daughter. Above all, I felt a real sense of self achievement, knowing that the greatest gift we can pass on to our children is the ability to live a healthy and happy lifestyle.

The Pram Diet tells the story of how I achieved this positive transformation and how every mum, everywhere, can too.

My Journey

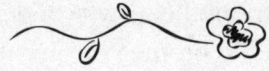

I have been asked many times, 'Have you always been self loving?' or 'Have you always been confident?'

The answer is **no**.

In fact, almost the opposite. Before discovering the vibrant lifestyle I call 'the pram diet', I had spent a great deal of my life ashamed of my body and overly judgemental of my appearance. Battling to keep my weight down, I was always critical of myself, always dissatisfied with my reflection in the mirror.

I believe that a lot of my issues with low self esteem and excess weight came from my childhood, as they do for many people. At primary school I was the object of peer teasing, and often compared myself unrealistically with images from the media. I developed unhealthy eating habits, unconsciously learning from people around me that one of the ways to deal with stress, anxiety, hurt and even happiness was to 'eat my emotions' – to comfort and reward myself with food. It is all too easy for someone such as I was, with low self esteem, to use 'treat' food as an emotional crutch, a way to feel good.

I grew up in a divorced family, with very loving households on both sides. My childhood was rich and full. I lived with my loving and attentive mother and adored spending time with my loving, caring father and amazing step-mother, my wonderful step-sisters, step-brothers and a brother on my mother's side as well. We moved house a few times but I always made friends easily, including boyfriends as I got older. Yet despite being a bright, imaginative and cheerful child I was often anxious about my appearance, a girl who, while a little overweight, imagined her reflection in the mirror to be so much bigger than it really was.

I wasn't always overweight, it yo-yoed a lot over the years when I was growing up. At times I had growth spurts and would slim right down, and I was always very active, riding my bike, walking to school and exploring the outdoors. But I was always eating, and eating a lot. Regardless of my actual size, I always felt overweight, unattractive and unfortunate looking, even when people tried to convince me otherwise.

When I was around eight or nine it was discovered that my vision was not as good as it should be. It felt to me then that I had really 'struck out in the genetic pool'. I was given glasses to wear, at first only for occasional use for long distance. It wasn't really an issue for me until I was around twelve and my eyesight became much worse. I could no longer read the blackboard well, I had trouble recognising people even at short distances and TV was becoming fuzzier by the day. Knowing full well what happens to the unfortunate ones who wear glasses at school and already considering myself to be at a great disadvantage because of my weight, I was not about to add the thickly rimmed and unattractive glasses to my image. I chose instead to try and make do, and my schooling suffered. About this time I started at a new high school in a different town and my struggles all seemed to slip under everybody's radar.

My personal despair had grown greatly, for my world and everything I loved to see was blurred. The more sadness and frustration I felt the more I put on a joking, lively personality to hide the real emotions at war within me.

At the age of thirteen I developed 'disruptive' behaviour in the classroom and would even skip school to avoid the embarrassment caused by my failing eyesight. I could not read the blackboard at all and, unnoticed in a large and bustling high school, I began to join the others who for their own personal reasons were not learning either. I lost the love of learning that had filled my childhood and for which I had always been known.

It was around this time that I met another girl obsessed with her weight. Even though I considered her to be gloriously slim and beautiful she devoted all her spare time to her appearance. I was no longer overweight for my age, but I vividly recalled from my childhood the pain and humiliation caused by chafing as my chubby legs rubbed together. I remembered having to sprinkle my thighs with talcum powder just so I could walk without pain in the heat of summer. Together my new friend and I ran every day, exercised for long periods and ate nothing but microwaved carrots with salt, some lettuce or occasionally a piece of grilled fish. Under her influence I lost more weight and my unhealthy lifestyle began to seriously affect my health and wellbeing. I developed real issues with food and was constantly concerned about my weight. I felt lower and more self conscious than ever.

At first it was just so exciting to have a kindred spirit who knew the pain and torment of hating your own appearance. It was such a deep relief to know that I was not alone. For a long time I wasted away, not eating for days at a time and when I did, eating very little and only things I considered non-fattening. I had become quite obsessed and never felt I was thin enough. At times I lived on chewing gum and cigarettes and I never felt happy or relaxed. I became so unhealthy that my hair felt thinner and dull and I began to get acne for the first time in my life. I suffered from constipation and the good, strong, straight white teeth I had been blessed with really took a beating. I felt short-tempered a lot, had frequent dizzy spells and could never seem to concentrate.

My self esteem was at an all-time low – I was convinced that I couldn't be thin enough and would cover up my tiny frame. I was never seen without a long jumper tied around my little waist to hide what I thought was my huge behind. I still could not stride confidently down the warm sands of a beautiful beach on a gloriously hot summer day in a two-piece bathing suit, but always swam in a baggy t-shirt and shorts.

At fifteen I was hospitalised with a very painful twisted fallopian tube and my mother was told by the specialist that I would probably never have children. I was devastated.

Despite all this, in my later teenage years I was fortunate enough to fall in love and be really cared for and appreciated, which did a great deal to help rebuild my confidence. But the care and attention never felt like enough and the restored confidence never seemed to last. Even so, I was able to return to studying at this time, an experience that brought me great happiness. My passionate love of learning met up with my fascination for plants and I enrolled in a horticulture course at college – it was a happy time indeed.

By the age of eighteen, though, my health was in a very bad state. I had constant chest infections, was anaemic and seemed to be forever getting ill. Desperate, I tried giving up smoking and started to eat again, not sensibly or healthily but returning to old, bad habits. In just four months I had put on a staggering amount of weight and wore the story of my weight fluctuations in tell-tale stretch marks. I felt like I was forever at war with the mirror.

At twenty-one I met Damien, the man who would be the love of my life and the father of my daughter. I thought I had known all manner of love but until I met him I didn't know that I could glow from pure happiness. He gave me strength and unconditional love and support, regardless of whatever size I was throughout my many failed attempts to lose the weight and keep it off. He taught me to see myself as beautiful and special, even if only through his eyes. Damien was already blessed with two beautiful children – a boy and a girl whom he loves dearly and who are both truly delightful.

It was around this time that I was fortunate enough to be employed at Bunnings Warehouse in Bundaberg. In this job I was given so much opportunity to develop, and to share my knowledge and love of plants. The management embraced my enthusiasm and creativity and really helped me to grow, not just careerwise but as an individual confident of my knowledge, skills and abilities and my capacity to work as a valued member of a team. I truly loved it. I loved the fulfilling and challenging experiences of maintaining, running, presenting and selling the plant nursery section. From this I created and ran my own successful garden club there, through which I was able to indulge my passion for writing by producing a garden club newsletter every month for Bunnings. I went on to present a gardening segment on a local community radio program and got involved in community events such as designing the Bunnings float for a town spring parade, and designing and organising plant displays for an agricultural show. My working life was full of exciting challenges that ensured I was using my creativity and knowledge on a daily basis. My home life was filled with love and happiness and as a couple we revelled in spending our weekends together, camping, exploring nature, sightseeing and generally having fun. During this busy and fulfilling time my self esteem was not an issue and the years seemed to pass very quickly.

Then, at twenty-four, I became ill. It was months before the cause of the problem was diagnosed as ovarian cysts. Meanwhile, there were many trips to the emergency department and to doctors, and a lot of time off work. Luckily I had an understanding employer who gave me as much time as I needed, a partner who was always there for me and my mother living close by. But the strain was intense. The pain was horrible. Sometimes it was like a hot stabbing knife and I would be momentarily frozen to the spot, other times it was a slow intense grinding pain that left me feeling crippled. It was a frustrating, painful, scary and desperate time of my life. Eventually, after many weeks, an ultrasound showed clusters of cysts on both ovaries, including a particularly large one on my right ovary which was causing the worst of the pain. The doctors debated whether to operate or take a more conservative approach to my treatment. I even narrowly escaped being a patient of the infamous Dr Patel or 'Dr Death' as he was later known, who was arranging for me to have exploratory surgery. Thankfully, a gynaecologist disagreed with him and sent me home instead with various medications, recommending this as the safest approach to treating ovarian cysts.

Throughout this time I was ill and in pain so often that I lost a lot of weight. So it was a slim me who at twenty-five discovered that I was going to be blessed with a baby. Damien and I were beside ourselves with excitement, blissfully and completely happy.

Mine was to be the very first 'Bunnings baby' for the Bundaberg store and the whole team supported me, celebrated my great news and shared in my excitement and joy as well as the delight at my growing belly. I felt very well cared for and looked after. I still had my exciting job, my loving and wonderful partner, Damien (by this stage my fiancé), and a beautiful baby to look forward to as well. I was brimming with happiness and really felt myself glow. I had no morning sickness and because I was pregnant, deliriously happy and had recently lost a lot of weight, I ate with wild abandon. I ate anything and everything I wanted to. I didn't care about calories, fat or quantities. I was constantly hungry and indulged every slight and single craving I had. I consumed very large quantities of all manner of food and the weight piled on. I didn't care. I convinced myself that the weight would just fall off once I had my baby. I believe people who knew me may have been shocked at how quickly I 'thickened' – but who would tell a pregnant woman she was eating too much? I felt starving all the time. The more I ate the more it seemed I wanted to eat and I eventually put on around 40 kilograms. This was most definitely not all baby and amniotic fluid.

I worked with so many wonderful people who all made my pregnancy feel really special. So many 'knew' Lily and talked to her daily when she was 'my bump'. Through the understanding and support of my employers and the team I worked with I was able to continue working and doing what I loved right through until almost the end of my pregnancy. This, combined with excellent care from the hospital midwives and devotion from Damien, helped to ensure that my days were busy, happy and exciting. My mother even moved into the granny flat at our house to help out with the coming baby.

Towards the end of my pregnancy, though, I became painfully constipated. I was extremely bloated and uncomfortable and my mood became irritable and short tempered. Looking back, I suspect that the years of eating processed foods and subjecting my body to crazy, unhealthy fad diets had caught up with me. I had never really stopped to consider the damage food could do to the inner workings of the body and back then, I wasn't really interested in finding out.

On 10 December 2005 at 9.45 am, after just four hours of labour, my daughter Lily was born. My labour was unexpectedly short and two weeks early, completely throwing out my detailed birth plan. I got to the hospital just an hour before Lily arrived and, assisted by our wonderful midwife, had a completely trouble-free natural birth. Four days later, we went home. After taking a couple of days off to help us settle in, my mother went back to work. Damien, Lily and I spent almost two beautiful and timeless weeks together before he also returned to work.

At first I relished the serenity and peace of being alone with Lily. I loved our precious time together and would often just sit and watch my baby, holding her close and listening to her soft breathing while she slept. I felt my heart would surely burst from such love. I couldn't believe how perfect she was and how much I adored her. Occasionally I even felt adventurous enough to escape the Queensland summer heat and take my new baby into the cool air-conditioned shopping centres. And of course we had to visit Bunnings so that everyone who had treated my 'bump' with such care and excitement could finally meet Lily.

I was still experiencing problems with constipation but tried not to think about it too much. Not all days were as bad as others but a really bad day, complete with sharp pains and intense bloating, was just awful. Constipation could make it difficult to enjoy outings and even to be comfortable sitting down.

After approximately two months we began having real troubles with Lily's feeding. It had never been really good but now it was becoming extremely painful and she seemed to be constantly wanting to feed. Every afternoon like clockwork she would cry for around an hour as I helplessly tried to console her. She would attach to my breast so strongly it felt as though my skin would tear, and she would always fall asleep during her feeds. My nipples became increasingly cracked, damaged and extremely painful. I remember one particular night of absolute agony when I lay in bed weeping with my baby hungrily feeding as I held my tear-soaked face into a pillow to prevent myself from screaming. I was a mess – possibly the most miserable and desperate I had ever felt. Damien could only look on helplessly as I cried my way through one of the worst nights of my life before he had to go off to work exhausted and emotionally drained.

The next day I went to see a doctor who advised using a nipple shield and treating the nipples with soothing ice packs as well as a prescribed cream. The alternative was to consider switching to a good formula. While I had nothing against formula, I wanted the very best for my child and was convinced that 'breast is best'. I felt that breastfeeding was one of the most important and natural aspects of being a mother so it was utterly distressing to be confronted with the possibility of giving it up when my daughter was still so young. I was on an emotional roller coaster of guilt, a sense of failure and frustration.

While visiting a chemist for yet another container of fibre drink to ease my clogged and painful bowels, I came across a baby check clinic and decided to get Lily checked over too. I felt so excited as she was weighed and measured until the nurse expressed concern that Lily wasn't gaining enough weight and referred us to a breastfeeding clinic. We had just assumed Lily was a slim baby because she was so very long – tallness is common in both our families. She fed regularly and was otherwise healthy, and as a new mother I didn't realise she wasn't getting enough sustenance from my milk.

The clinic confirmed she was not putting on enough weight and the nurse explained that Lily hadn't been suckling properly all this time. She also explained that I wasn't producing enough milk. When Lily was born she was 'tongue tied', which had caused some initial feeding difficulties until that problem was fixed. Now it was discovered that our technique together wasn't very good and that she was having lots of little feeds, as opposed to a few good long deep ones. I was so sorry I hadn't known about the clinic earlier.

After fervently expressing to the nurse my absolute determination to breastfeed I was encouraged to buy a breast pump and begin expressing between feeds, to try and increase my milk supply. Due to very restricted finances we were only able to acquire a manual pump which was exhausting and uncomfortable to use, yet I was so determined to do the right thing for my baby that I persevered. When it was obvious this approach wasn't working I began taking herbal remedies and supplements that the nurse had also recommended, building up my hopes only to have them shattered miserably when nothing worked. I finally concluded that I was obviously a failure and must not be a natural mother. My own mother, while always trying to help and give good advice, seemed to be constantly telling me how well she had breastfed my brother and myself. In the end I felt I was letting her down as well as my daughter when, on medical advice, I began to supplement my baby's feeds each day with one of the recommended formulas. Once Lily discovered the ease of feeding from a bottle she began to need real encouragement and coaxing to take the breast at all, and I remember on some occasions her crying at the mere sight of it. I was still expressing at every opportunity and my breasts were extremely sore. I was utterly exhausted.

I felt such a mess. I felt defeated. I felt a failure. I felt tired beyond belief. I felt like a bad mother and I felt very depressed and despairing. I also felt keenly the lack of conversation, stimulation, friendship, laughter, responsibilities and challenges that had previously been a core part of my daily life. I felt slower, sluggish and unmotivated. My opinion was no longer sought, my knowledge quite unnecessary, my time not important. I felt isolated and friendless. I imagined my years of study becoming worthless, my knowledge fading away and my thought processes fogging over and becoming duller with each passing day. I loved my baby so completely yet I also felt torn, no longer cared about or important to anyone but my beautiful baby who would one day be all grown up. I remember, around this time, telling my mother how overweight and unattractive I felt, to which she well-meaningly replied, 'It really doesn't matter how you look anyway, you're a mum now'. She was trying to be supportive, but her comment devastated me all the same.

In my depressed state I saw the person who was me as a completely failed 'mum' figure. I felt very one dimensional. I felt I was letting my daughter down. I was drowning in a world of sleepless nights, feeding problems, an unhappy baby, financial strains, painful bloating, no energy, endless washing, neverending housework, chores and cleaning, constant worrying, no real conversation and such a sense of failure.

I felt I was under so much pressure to be a perfect mother and homemaker even though I really had no such expectations from my partner or anyone else – they all came from me. As my problems increased I reacted by obsessively cleaning, cooking, washing and trying desperately to be a perfect housewife. I would collapse exhausted, ashamed and defeated at the end of every day. My one indulgence was the time I spent alone in my nightly shower. I had always worked or studied. Now, staying at home with my baby had reduced us to the financial strain of trying to live on one income. On top of everything else, I felt immense guilt about this. Every time bills came in and payments were due my sense of guilt returned and I would work myself even harder. I never seemed to sit down or relax – there was always something to be done.

My depression felt like a living thing that grew

with each passing day. I was far too ashamed to admit to myself that I might have post-natal depression, let alone seek the help I so desperately needed. It was only later that I discovered how supportive, non-judgemental and caring other mothers, doctors, nurses and relevant organisations are and the great relief and help they can give you.

To my exhausted, despairing state I began adding disappointment in myself whenever I caught a glimpse of my reflection and all the excess, sagging weight I carried. I saw the stretch marks not as the result of creating a beautiful life but rather as an addition to my ugliness and sorry sense of self. I felt alone and didn't let anyone in, although I always put on a brave and happy face. I began to avoid being in family photos or would cut myself out of them. I couldn't bear to see the way I looked and I didn't want my precious daughter to remember me that way. I was irrational, oversensitive, on edge all the time, putting huge and unrealistic pressure on myself. I wasn't sleeping properly, and ground my teeth in my sleep. All this must have been truly awful for Damien to live with, but he did, patiently, supportively and without complaint or question. For this I am forever grateful.

PRAM WALKING

Eventually, one day, I reached breaking point. I could cry no more. I had had enough.

Angry and frustrated, I bundled my baby into her pram and packed it with every conceivable thing I could possibly need or want, and then some. Once I was sure Lily was comfortable and safe in the pram, well shielded from the burning sun and protected from the wind, we set off stormily on a long life-changing walk.

It was this moment, this walk, that would change my life forever.

I returned from this rejuvenating and exhilarating walk a new version of myself. The pram that I had only ever viewed as a burdensome, awkward and heavy contraption was now a treasured tool, a means of escape from the ill feelings I was brooding on. It offered a fantastic workout that I could, most importantly, do *with my baby*, working my muscles as I pushed it along. It enabled me to get out into that precious, revitalising fresh air and the walk left me feeling utterly alive, inspired and excited. I could hardly wait for the next day to do it all over again.

There would be no turning back.

As Lily and I took our daily pram walks together, each week the distance got longer and longer and my depression got less and less. I was realistic, starting with short routes and being careful not to overdo it, let it become boring or make the walk into a chore. At first I walked around two blocks or so of my neighbourhood; then, as my fitness improved, I gradually increased the distance until we were comfortably walking about five kilometres (one to one-and-a-half hours) five times a week. I felt so good that I started finding extra walking opportunities in everyday tasks whenever I could.

I was enjoying my life a little more each day and worrying over the small things a little less. I felt my clothing becoming looser on me as I began to feel fitter, less tired and more in control of my life and my emotions. When I had first begun walking, I was overweight, wearing loose baggy clothes and back to sprinkling talcum powder on my thighs to prevent them rubbing together painfully on those hot, humid Queensland days. I would never have considered wearing shorts. But after only a few months, my skirts were so loose I couldn't hold them up, even with a belt, and I realised to my delight that I didn't need the talcum powder any more. Now I wear shorts often.

My baby loved her pram and the soothing motion as we walked along. She would listen happily to my voice as I chatted or sang to her when she was awake. And when the relaxing rhythm lulled her to sleep I loved to watch her as I walked.

I realised that if it was this easy to lose weight, to feel so much fitter and so much less stressed, my pram walking regime would be easy to maintain. I felt as though the lights had been switched back on.

As the weight came off and I started feeling really good I began to look at my diet. The more I looked the more I saw how unhealthy it was. I realised I wasn't eating nearly enough fibre, let alone fruit and vegetables. I was acutely aware that if I wanted my daughter to eat healthy fresh foods I needed to change my own diet first.

I really began to embrace 'fresh is best', and to eat more natural foods, whole grains, fruit snacks and foods high in antioxidants. I also made sure I drank at least eight big glasses of water every day.

The less sugar-laden foods I ate, the less sugary foods I craved. In fact, some highly processed foods began to make me feel a little ill because they were so artificially sweet or greasy. I never felt deprived or hungry; in fact, I actually began to want the healthy options. I went looking for information about foods that improve health and wellbeing, gradually adding to my list of foods items that had particular benefits, were especially nutritious, or high in fibre or particular nutrients. I was developing a whole new appreciation of healthy foods, realising how delicious they can taste.

I was amazed at just how easy it was to make small changes in our day-to-day eating habits and family meals, changes that could produce such significant health benefits for all of us. I started bulking out our evening meals with lots of steamed fresh veggies and fresh tasty salads. I stopped eating as soon as I felt full, served my meals on a smaller dinner plate, ate breakfast from a smaller cereal bowl, and read the labels carefully on any processed foods I ate. These kinds of simple changes made such a difference to my health. Each small change would lead to another, always feeling achievable, yet building to a major lifestyle change that brought enormous benefits.

The combination of daily exercise, drinking lots of water and eating high-fibre and healthy foods began to ease my constipation. My body was starting to function efficiently again and I felt refreshed and re-energised. In fact, I felt inspired, and proud that I was finally accessing the inner strength I had never previously been able to acknowledge.

The cost and quality of fresh fruit and vegetables can be a huge factor at the supermarket, particularly when you want to go for the very best and eat organic, so I decided after a while that I would put my horticultural knowledge to good use. Despite the obstacles – we were renting, the gardens had poor soil, we had two dogs who were going to trample any young plants, and our budget was tight – I started growing our own fresh organic fruit and vegetables. It took a creative approach and it turned out to be a lot of fun. Along with the pram walking, it was one of the best decisions of my life.

Growing our own produce was wonderfully rewarding and gave me back that stimulation and creativity I had been missing so much. Best of all, my baby loved it too. Lying on a soft blanket in the shade next to me or in her cosy pram, she loved listening to the lively sounds of birds, the wind, the outdoors all around her. I wanted to be a positive role model for my daughter and teach her invaluable life lessons about healthy foods – what better way than to involve her in growing our own fruit and vegetables?

Gardening is such a revitalising thing to do – being out in the glorious, fresh air, being in touch with nature and feeling the raw earth between your fingers and the satisfaction of nurturing, feeding and watering young plants. I felt such delight and pride in harvesting our very own fresh produce and creatively cooking it into tasty, healthy meals. It was so reassuring to know everything that had happened to the vegetables I puréed into organic baby foods for Lily. And seeing the grocery bill come down as the producing garden provided more and more of our food was an inspiring bonus.

The love and appreciation of cooking has always been around me. My grandmother was an accomplished chef. My mother worked for years as a professional cook and a chef, running a boutique café when I was growing up. And my step-mother was a brilliant and talented cook, too, capable of great feats in the kitchen. Applying this love of cooking to healthy, fresh ingredients really helped me make the most of wholesome foods and healthy eating. At first, my fiancé was alarmed at the thought of eating low-fat 'healthy' cooking, but once he started sampling the revamped meals and baked goodies he was delighted and enjoyed eating the foods as much I enjoyed making them.

My life had changed. I felt fantastic. I felt lighter. I felt freer and I felt more alive, happier than I could ever remember – and the results spoke for themselves. I had lost over 28 kilos but I had also gained muscle, fitness, confidence and excitement in every day, and had a whole new lease on life.

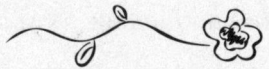

These days, I can confidently and proudly watch my toddler picking fresh snow peas, munching on a stalk of celery straight from the garden, excitedly running to the hanging strawberry baskets to check for any red ones, or asking for a 'treat' of cherry tomatoes when we go shopping. I love the way she helps in our gardens, learning about the frogs and plants, marvelling at a praying mantis nest covered in a hundred babies that are pretending not to be seen, or watching the butterflies visit the flowers. And I love to see her edgy with excitement when we go to the local community farmers' markets to buy fresh produce, then relaxing in her stroller, contentedly eating whatever fruit is in season.

We continue to take our daily walks, with Lily in a stroller now. I feel full of life and can enjoy and fully relish the experience of a family outing to the beach. And I feel such inner peace, such relief from all the pain and sadness I had so unnecessarily carried inside me for so long.

People who knew me before remark on how great I look, the amazing difference in me, how I seem so radiant and beautiful. I have finally come to understand what it is that makes a person truly beautiful – that confidence, happiness, love of self and love of life can really make you shine.

It has been a long and winding path of learning, loving, being loved and letting go . . .

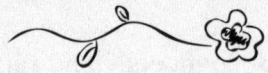

In the rest of this book I share with you, dear reader, what I have discovered on my journey to good health, happiness and living well. By making the small changes I suggest, by taking these positive steps and believing in yourself, I hope you too will walk the path to a healthier and happier you.

Nurturing Your Self

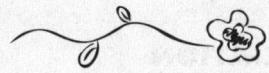

Until I started living the combination of lifestyle choices that make up the pram diet, much of my life revolved around struggling with weight issues and low self esteem. Once I transformed my lifestyle, however, my view of myself changed radically.

One mantra that has helped me enormously is this: *The very best person to be is the very best version of myself.*

From my own experience I know it is possible to have extremely low self esteem or a low sense of self worth, yet still appear to function very well. It is often assumed that if you have low self esteem or 'don't really like who you are', you will be a withdrawn kind of person. But that is not always the case. You can even be considered 'lively' and 'funny' and 'warm' by people who know and love you, and those qualities might make up a significant part of your personality, but in the deeper reaches of yourself, the emotional and feeling part of you, there can lurk a deep sadness that is a low sense of self. There were times when I seemed fine, yet would stand in front of the mirror and hear these words in my head: 'I looked into the mirror and what did I see? A great wave of negativity directed at me'.

SELF APPRECIATION

To look at your own reflection without judgement, without criticism, without shame, without guilt, without comparing yourself negatively to others or to media-driven ideals is one of the greatest accomplishments a woman can achieve.

As women we are typically the care givers, peace keepers, nurturers and the loving warm hearts of our families.

Yet how often do we stand back and take the time to appreciate ourselves – everything we do, everything we give, everything we have achieved, and how skilful and special we really are? We frequently underestimate ourselves, rarely giving ourselves credit for our many achievements both personal and practical.

The path to success lies in believing in ourselves, in nurturing our dreams and in having the heart, self appreciation, dignity and self respect to follow them.

Some of the greatest success stories and most dramatic achievements feature seemingly 'ordinary' people who have believed in themselves and followed their dreams.

Being happy is considered a strong indicator of success, so it follows that we need to discover and pursue what makes us happy if we are to lead truly successful, fulfilling lives. We are all special, with unique qualities, abilities, personalities and passions. Yet finding and nurturing a strong, resilient sense of self does not always come naturally. Many of us need to learn or relearn how to believe in ourselves, to view ourselves kindly with appreciation, dignity and respect, and to acknowledge how special we are.

Only you know what makes you deeply happy, what your secret dreams and passions are. But the following checklist might help make it easier for you to stay on track in your pursuit of self appreciation:

- believe in yourself
- follow your dreams
- listen with your heart
- be grateful for the blessings in your life
- be open to new possibilities
- accept warmth and love when it is freely given
- give love openly and unconditionally
- accept compliments sincerely when they are offered genuinely
- know that you deserve to be happy every day
- turn every thought into a positive one
- see the good in everything and everyone

- take the time sometimes just to 'be'
- let go of needing to understand and control every-thing
- look forward rather than dwelling on the past
- be true to yourself

Inner beauty

Real, breathtaking, empowering beauty is a reflection of true happiness and always comes from within. Inner beauty is something that cannot be faked. It cannot be created, not even by the best plastic surgeons in the world; it doesn't come from designer labels and it has no relevance to income, age, the street you live in, or where you come from.

It is a glow – a radiant, beautiful glow – that envelops a person with a presence and confidence that touches and inspires everyone who comes near. Inner beauty comes from your heart and your mind. It shines in your eyes, it tickles your mouth into an endless smile.

Inner beauty is awe inspiring and contagious. It reflects a strength of character that will help you through difficult times, give you the capacity to achieve what you really want, and energise you with the drive and motivation to reach for your goals. It sustains a sense of pride and self respect. It comes from loving who you are and everything you are, and from striving to be the very best that you can be. It is founded on a belief that you deserve to be happy, appreciated, respected and loved. Especially by yourself.

Inner beauty recognises the image in your mirror as the amazing, talented, worthy, beautiful woman you truly are. It lends lightness and bounce to every step you take, regardless of the destination. It allows you to greet each day with a smile and a feeling of excitement at the possibilities a new day brings.

We are so much more than the physical image of ourselves – we are our thoughts, our dreams, our hopes, our kindness, our loves and our goals. When we deeply believe in ourselves, believe in our inner strengths and our unique abilities, we tap into our inner beauty and discover the capacity for achieving success in every aspect of our lives.

There is a direct link between feeling good and being inspired by ourselves for ourselves to be all that we can be – to be role models for our children, to be real women with real goals and real confidence in ourselves; to want to look after ourselves and have genuine pride in our reflection; to take good care of ourselves both physically emotionally, to be happy both inside and out. When we tap into our inner beauty we know that we are worth the effort, that we all deserve to be happy, healthy, fit and active, feeling fantastic and full of energy each and every day.

The greatest gift we can give ourselves, our families, our friends and loved ones is our inner beauty shining through.

OVERCOMING NEGATIVITY AND STRESS

A negative mood can envelop you like a heavy shawl. When you are feeling down or depressed, children, especially babies and toddlers, will pick up on your feelings and can often become restless, irritable, cranky and unable to sleep peacefully. Older children might exhibit naughty or sulky behaviours and you might also find yourself arguing with your partner and loved ones over the smallest things. All this will result in you feeling even worse.

When you are feeling negative it seems almost impossible to do anything to help yourself, or to overcome the problems and issues that pervade your life. Yet one of the most effective things you can do at times like this is to work at discovering your inner beauty. When you're in the depths of gloom, self appreciation might seem like a pointless exercise, but if you focus on the attributes and attitudes listed on page 29, you are likely to find yourself feeling more positive, happier and more optimistic. Focusing on inner beauty might not instantly resolve or remove all your problems, but it will bring countless benefits to you and your family as the quality of your day-to-day life and your overall health improves.

Relentless negativity causes damaging stress for you and your family, and stress can wreak havoc in your life. In short, sharp bursts, stress is a constructive force that triggers a primal survival mechanism, heightening the senses and intensifying reactions, enabling a creature under threat to take flight, to defend their young, or to burst into a ferocious attack on prey. But on a prolonged basis, stress can have damaging effects on the physical body as well as the mind.

Training yourself to be more positive, along with getting out and getting active, is one of the most effective ways of reducing stress. Once you view your life through a positive lens you will be able to see and activate a whole range of other stress-relieving lifestyle choices.

Start by concentrating on what is good in your life – it's all too easy to get caught up in what we don't have, can't do or would like to change. Remember, there is always someone else who has less than you have and who is doing it harder.

Try writing a list of what you do have, taking time to be grateful for people and things you might normally take for granted. Appreciate the positives in yourself and in your situation, and in the people who might seem at times to be part of the problem. You might give it a heading like 'Gratitude list' or 'Things I appreciate in my life right now'.

Your gratitude list might include:

- family members who love you
- your children
- your home
- support networks
- community resources
- friends

- sentimental items
- personal treasures
- your talents and skills
- your favourite physical feature
- your lovable qualities and positive attributes
- your personal achievements (becoming a mum is a huge one!)

The more time you spend on compiling this list, the more you remind yourself of the positives in your life and how fortunate you are to have them.

Once you have developed your gratitude list, it will be easier to generate positive thoughts that help to improve your mood. Make them as personal as you like.

Here are some general suggestions for positive self-talk:

- I'm a mum – how wonderful is that!
- I have such a beautiful family.
- I have had a really constructive day today.
- I'm going to treat myself to a relaxing bath tonight once the kids are in bed.
- I really am fortunate with the things I have in my life.
- I really enjoyed my walk today and I am looking forward to the walk tomorrow.
- How beautiful the weather is today!
- I have really great friends.
- My garden is coming along very well.
- I am feeling healthier every day.

- I am a talented and successful person.
- I have done some amazing things in my life.

Make a conscious effort to start your day thinking positive and feeling fresh. Put your gratitude list somewhere easy to see, and refer to it often. Focus on small and big positives and every small and big thing that makes you feel good. And always let your last thoughts as you drift off to sleep be pleasant and positive ones. It won't be long before you are looking for ways to bring more positives into your life.

PRAM WALKING AND OTHER MOOD LIFTERS

Focusing on inner beauty, gratitude and positive thoughts are just some of the ways you can start to dissolve negativity and gloom. Physical exercise is another key part of the program. In fact, if you struggle with changing your attitude, then take your pram (and baby) for a walk instead, and you'll soon find that positive thoughts come more easily. Exercise releases endorphins in the brain – and endorphins are the brain chemicals that tell us we are happy and feeling fine.

Remember, the pram diet all began when I got fed up with feeling depressed and strode off with my baby for a life-changing walk. Here are some simple ideas that will help you dispel stress and negativity once and for all:

- **Go for a walk!** Put your little one in the pram, pack it up with everything you could possibly need and get out in that fresh air. Enjoy the boost of feel-good endorphins! This is the best stress relief you are likely to find – and it's free. It has always worked for me regardless of how bad I felt, how tired I was or how upset I had been. Pram walking was the one thing that could instantly make me feel better every single time.

- **Breathing.** Step aside from whatever stressful situation you find yourself in, and calmly relax your whole body by taking a big deep slow breath. Let the breath out again really slowly (close your eyes if that helps). Once you have repeated this several times you will find the tension and stress have eased.

- **Drink lots of water.** Pour yourself a really big glass of water. If you like, add some slices of fresh lemon and some ice blocks, sit down and take the time to enjoy drinking it.

- **Take a virtual break.** Cut out a picture of your ideal holiday destination or an image of a place that looks relaxing (even if you've never been there). Keep the picture handy for those stressful moments. When stress or negativity creep in, take a few minutes to gaze deeply into the image and really feel yourself there, without a care in the world. Even if you only do this for a half a minute or so, it can be a surprisingly powerful mood lifter.

- **Tone your body.** Use your frustration to power you through a set of ten mini push-ups, sit-ups or squats.
- **Go gardening.** Take a shovel and churn up some dirt in the backyard. Dig up the soil where you want your veggie patch to be. The physical exertion will soon dissolve your stress and negativity.
- **Sit with nature.** Go outside with your little one and just sit for a moment with them. See the world through their eyes, observe the magic of life and the true beauty of nature that is around us all the time. Clear your head and feel yourself totally present, experiencing with your child's awe the sheer delight that is life.
- **Journey to the stars.** At night, take a few minutes to go outside and stare in wonder at the magnitude and grandeur of the stars and the night sky. To experience the full impact of this nocturnal journey, lie down somewhere quiet and dark. If you have older children, involve them in the experience and gaze at the great wonder of the night sky together.
- **Scrub and clean.** It might sound strange but cleaning can actually be very therapeutic. Try giving your bathroom or laundry a thorough scrubbing and cleaning, then enjoy the freshness of it and the feeling of achievement.

These are activities I have found to be really effective in relieving stress and tension. For me, going for a walk with my baby daughter in the pram, enjoying the fresh air and distractions of being outside, was the ultimate mood-lifting experience. It offered me a free and invigorating escape from the endless monotony of the household chores. And it shifted my perspective, reminding me that I am a tiny, tiny piece in the grand puzzle that is life, and that my problems, even when they seem all-consuming, can be resolved.

FOOD FOR THOUGHT

The human body is truly extraordinary. It is capable of great feats of athleticism, endurance and performance. It can be shaped and toned so well with the techniques, knowledge and equipment that are now readily available to us. Why, then, are so many of us unhappy with our physical reflection in the mirror? Why are many of us not fully utilising and maintaining the magnificent body each of us has?

What is it that drives us to eat unhealthily? When we know it is not good for us, why do we reach for that whole block of chocolate, that large serve of chips, the ice cream straight from the container, the pizza, the huge dinner portions? Why do we head for the drive-through takeaway instead of making a healthy salad?

How many of the following statements do you relate to? I am unhappy with my body. I obsess about food. I am frustrated with the image that looks back at me in the mirror. I yo-yo from one crazy diet to another. I'm always thinking about my weight, what I'm going to eat next or what I've just eaten. I'm concerned about how I look and how others might see me.

Once you decide that you have already spent too much of your life angsting about food and self image, if your life is not full of the joy and zing and self confidence you want for yourself, it is time to start looking at the self image you really want and what you need to do to achieve it.

If your body is not looking its fittest and trimmest, chances are you could also be feeling sluggish and low in energy, finding it hard to keep up with your children and being short of breath after light exercise or a gentle walk. Perhaps you have begun pram walking, or other kinds of physical exercise. A food review might be the next item on your self nurture list.

How, what and why do you eat?

How many times have you eaten past your full point and felt uncomfortable or even slightly ill afterwards? How often have you eaten something – maybe even a whole meal – when you weren't feeling hungry at all, but it was just there, or it was offered to you?

When was the last time you heard your stomach rumble or remember feeling genuinely hungry before a meal?

In this fortunate part of the world, buying, preparing and eating food are integral aspects of every day. Food, healthy and not so healthy, is readily available. Why, then, is it such a problematic issue for so many women? Why do we compromise our health with erratic or poor food choices, especially when our family's health and happiness relies on us being fit and happy and well?

Why is it that an ever-busy mother will prepare wholesome foods and packed lunches for her family but grab 'whatever' from the cupboard, fridge or local shop when it comes to feeding herself? Why are we so skilled at providing our children and families with all the right vitamins and minerals but can't always be bothered when it comes to ourselves?

And why do we encourage our children to be active and involved in sports, only to sit back and watch, or get on with our work, as they ride their bikes, go swimming or play a game of cricket? When was the last time you went out and had some active fun with the family or tried something new and challenging for yourself like golf, rollerblading, bushwalking, netball, jogging, water aerobics, yoga or swimming?

When was the last time you fell into bed feeling truly and wonderfully tired from a day's healthy exercise?

Eating our emotions

For many women, especially those who are mothers of young children, there is a real resistance to the idea of taking care of ourselves, or spending time and effort on improving our physical and emotional health, wellbeing and lifestyle. Many of us resist giving to ourselves the love, care and attention we openly and generously give to our families. Some of us simply put our own needs so far down the list that they are never properly addressed. And for some women, there can be real feelings of guilt associated with devoting time or energy to nurturing the self.

One solution to this dilemma involves 'eating our emotions' – turning to food as a quick, readily available pick-me-up or reward to support us through the day when we are busy devoting time and energy to the needs of everybody else.

How do you know if you are engaging in emotional eating? If you reach for food at the first sign of a stressful situation, bad or upsetting news, the arrival of a bill in the mail, a disappointment, or at times when you are feeling unappreciated or unloved, then you are probably in the habit of eating for comfort. Yet eating like this never solves our problems. Nor does it really make us feel all that much better. In fact, it can often make us feel even worse, adding guilt and unwanted kilograms to whatever stress or distress we were already feeling.

We don't even have to be feeling stressed or unappreciated to use food as an emotional prop. Many of us 'treat' ourselves when we run errands in town or catch up with friends. We enjoy a 'little food reward' because we have had a good day, received a pleasing report, achieved a goal or completed all our housework for the day.

Boredom can be another trigger for overeating. Sometimes, when we aren't being stimulated intellectually, creatively, imaginatively or physically we can spend big chunks of our days searching for something extra, something to stimulate us or create a temporary distraction from the boredom. It's all too easy, in these circumstances, to turn to food.

Occasionally, we can even eat out of fear – fear of rejection, fear of failure, fear of being attractive, fear of coming to terms with a truly awful personal experience or something from our past. This can be one of the hardest causes of emotional eating to overcome because we are, in a sense, 'hiding' ourselves under a perceived protective layer of excess weight.

The habit of comforting or rewarding ourselves with food is one we can unwittingly pass on to our children. In fact, our own parents may very well have accidentally passed it down us.

Eating for life

When we begin to look at why we overeat we start seeing patterns, recognising learned bad habits and, often, discovering suppressed issues of low self esteem or other damaging emotions. The path to understanding and overcoming these triggers is not always easy, but the rewards can be life-changing.

The good news is – we don't have to deal with all the issues and challenges in one go. The journey to good health and a fulfilling, vibrant, active lifestyle starts with just one step, just one decision, just one thought. Deciding to create positive change puts us on a path to increased awareness, an improved quality of life, a new level of happiness, health, fun and wellbeing and, most importantly, a strong sense of self.

Developing a good relationship with *all* foods is one major step along the path. It is so important to understand the pros and cons of everything you eat, and to choose foods that provide you with a *balanced* diet. It's okay to eat small quantities of 'unhealthy' foods occasionally so long as they are balanced out by the other foods you eat and the exercise you do. Feeling guilty about eating one ice cream on a family outing, or one square of good quality dark chocolate, leads you straight back into an emotional relationship with food – which is not something you want to include in your new, healthy way of life.

The following pages outline a wide range of techniques and strategies that can help you develop a new and healthy relationship with food. Many of these I discovered on my own journey to wellness and happiness – from personal experience, I know how effective they can be. And it's not always about food. There are lots of ideas about ways you can nurture and indulge yourself without involving food in the equation.

I also learned that once you've established a sensible eating regime you actually end up snacking less, even though sometimes you feel as though you are eating more. If, like me, you cringe at the thought of a heavy breakfast, then something like the Watermelon Smoothie (page 156) or the Exotic Holiday Yogurt (page 148) is perfect. Even munching on some fresh fruit pieces drizzled with fresh passionfruit will get your day off to a great start.

One of the best things I learned is to eat well before going grocery shopping – if necessary, take a packed lunch and eat it before you go anywhere near the supermarket. You will not only shop more cost effectively – you will also be much less tempted to drop sugary snacks, pre-packaged meals and calorie-laden 'food treats' into your trolley.

When you develop a healthy relationship with food, you discover the pleasure in savouring fresh natural tastes and textures, the satisfaction of preparing healthy, nourishing meals and sharing them with family and friends. You will no longer be tempted to eat for eating's sake, or for comfort or emotional support. You will be well on your way to discovering the benefits of a healthy, active lifestyle and strong self esteem.

SELF-NURTURING REWARDS AND TREATS

By now you will know that I consider a good long walk or a slice of luscious watermelon to be wonderfully rewarding treats. There are so many simple ways of nurturing yourself. Even personal treats you might once have considered unjustifiable or too expensive can be added to the list. If you keep track of the money you would previously have spent on snacks and takeaway food, you will be astonished at how quickly it adds up. You can put it towards 'extras' for the family, as well as the occasional 'indulgence' for yourself.

Here are some ideas to trigger your imagination:

- **Treat your trusty feet,** often the most neglected part of the body. Give them a five- to ten-minute soothing soak in warm water to which you have added a few drops of lavender essential oil. Dry them with a soft fluffy towel. Trim and buff your toenails. Then, if you like, finish them off with a fresh coat of a new nail polish in a colour that you love.
- **Lie in the shade or morning sun** for five to fifteen minutes, all by yourself.
- **Visit a health food store** and try some new natural skincare and haircare products.
- If you've had a particularly hard day or week, why not **treat yourself to an interesting magazine or book**?
- **A self-administered five-minute facial,** a green clay mask and cucumber slices over the eyes is an age-old traditional beauty regime. Lie down in a quiet place for five minutes and let your mind and body relax. It really does leave you feeling wonderful.
- **Visit a fresh fruit and vegetable store or market** and treat yourself to some of the more exotic or unusual fruits.

- **Visit a shop that specialises in herbs and spices** and have a chat to an expert about what you might like to try and how they are used. Herbs and spices can add flavour and interest to a wide range of healthy meals, doing away with the need to add salt, sugar or fats. (By the way, the less of these you consume, the less you crave or want.)

- **Buy yourself some quality kitchen utensils** that make healthy eating easier or food preparation quicker.

- **Visit your local video store or library** and borrow some DVDs purely for your own enjoyment. Or borrow a book you've been meaning to read.

- **Take your little one somewhere you would really like to visit,** and go for a scenic walk together. There are so many interesting places that are great backdrops for a walk, picnic and play with your baby, toddler or older child. Most botanic gardens, national parks, rainforest walks, oceanfronts and riversides have paths where you can walk with a pram or stroller. Or you can make a day of it and explore a small nearby town or village, a wildlife park or the zoo. Consider inviting some other mums and children along, to make it a really enjoyable social outing as well.

- **Have some 'silly time'!** Just yourself and your little one, playing in the backyard. Follow your child's lead and be carefree – let everything else wait.

- **Set up a medium- to long-term system of goals and rewards for yourself.** For example, a week-long goal might be to eat healthily and go for a walk every day. If you meet that goal, reward yourself with a new accessory, magazine, book, nail polish or other small item. If you've done well all month, your reward might be something more substantial like that dress you've had your eye on, a new bottle of perfume, a trip to the movies, paying for someone to clean your house, a massage, a family fun day of your choosing, a makeover, a visit to the hairdresser's – let your imagination loose.

- **Reward yourself with your favourite music.** Download some songs or buy that CD.
- **Have a bath.** If your home has a bathtub, treat yourself to a deep warm relaxing bath. Add bubbles, perfumed essential oils or bath salts to suit your mood. Make the room as dark as possible, and light a candle to enhance the relaxing atmosphere.
- **Take a night off from cooking.** Prepare a healthy meal like quiche and a sweet potato salad the day before, and store it well so the next night's dinner is taken care of. If you have older children or a partner who likes to cook, have them choose a healthy, nutritious recipe as their signature dish. Designate one night a week, or a fortnight, as your official night off and let the other family members take turns in the kitchen.
- **Visit your local plant nursery** and choose a delightful plant to liven up your home. Indoor plants have long been known to help purify the air and remove toxins, so why not improve the air

you and your family breathe with a hardy non-toxic indoor plant or two?

- **Start redecorating a room in your home,** one item at a time. For example, if you decide to give your bathroom a makeover, choose a colour scheme and theme. Then, each week (or fortnight, or month) when you meet your health and fitness goals, reward yourself by buying one item to go with your new look. Finances permitting, you could start with something big like painting the walls or buying a complete set of matching towels. Even new toothbrushes, a hand towel, bathmat or soap holder will make a surprising difference. Seeing the gradual transformation of your room provides a real incentive each week to keep going with your personal transformation.

- **Be creative.** Spend half an hour painting, knitting, scrapbooking, drawing, writing, quilting, designing, jewellery making, sewing. Even if you're not particularly skilled or experienced at arts or crafts, the very act of 'adult play' helps relieve tension, shift your focus and recharge your batteries.

- **Join a club or group.** As a big reward for doing well for a whole month or reaching a major goal, sign up with a club you've always been interested in. It could be a sewing group, a gardening club, a local wildlife organisation, a book club, a scrapbooking group, a theatre group or a choir – whatever appeals to you. If you find it hard getting to meetings you can still enjoy membership benefits like newsletters, special offers, merchandise, magazines and major events or outings. Special interest clubs and groups are a great way to meet people with similar interests to your own and enjoy some stimulating adult conversation.

- **Plan a holiday.** Set a goal so that if you walk every day and eat healthily consistently for, say, three, six or twelve months you will take your new, healthy, active self (and partner and family) on a relaxing holiday. Start saving when you start your new lifestyle plan and watch the fund grow as you transform!

CREATIVITY

Creative and artistic expression is a great tool for releasing tension, stress, frustrations and anxiety. Creative and artistic activity lets you unwind and relax while also stimulating your mind. Even if you've never been particularly gifted at arts and crafts, or interested in artistic pursuits, it doesn't mean you can't enjoy the therapeutic benefits they bring. In our society's stressful and demanding lives, finding a creative outlet far removed from the routine of our everyday lives is really worth the effort.

Hobbies and activities that allow you to use your imagination, gain new skills, freely express yourself in a creative way and exercise your mind can not only ground you but give you a sense of pride and achievement.

They even help with monitoring 'emotional eating'. Depending on the type of creative activity decide on, you can use your hobby to keep you busy at night when the children have gone to bed. Reward yourself with creative activity instead of snacking on lollies, chips and ice cream.

Once you put your mind to it, there are so many possibilities to choose from. You may already have a creative hobby that you never seem to have time for, or a long-forgotten artistic pastime you once enjoyed and would like to revisit. If you're not sure where to start, the best way is to try several activities before committing to any particular one, especially if your time or resources are limited. Your chosen activity should be one that invigorates and stimulates you.

Here are a few ideas to get you thinking:

- painting and drawing
- woodworking and model making
- jewellery making
- sewing and needlework
- knitting or crochet
- photography
- seed collecting and flower pressing
- playing musical instruments
- singing (consider joining a choir)
- pottery
- sculpting
- jigsaw puzzles
- clothing designs and creations

- cake cooking and decorating
- garden design and plant propagation
- flower arranging and floristry
- making preserves, jams and pickles
- dancing, performing, acting and taking lessons in these areas
- writing, song writing and poetry
- puzzles and crosswords
- scrapbooking
- candle making

It is a field of endless possibilities once you put your imagination to it.

While it can be difficult finding the time you need for your creative outlet, giving it importance and scheduling it into your routine will make that task much easier.

Unleashing your creative and artistic self will help you feel more relaxed, fulfilled and generally entertained in life. As your children grow older, you may be able to include them in your creative pursuits, sharing and passing on skills.

Creating your own special place

Having a place, however small, that is your own personal space can be like an oasis in the hurly-burly of family life. A special place can be anywhere, from a whole room to an outdoor area, a seat in the garden or a small corner of your home.

Where and how you create your special space will be up to you, the options you have and whatever epitomises a calming, tranquil setting to you. For some it will always be somewhere in the garden – basking in the sunlight among beds of happy flowers, a hammock hanging beneath a mighty tree, a corner on the patio with a table and chairs or a secret retreat in the soothing shade. Others will find theirs inside the home – an aromatic bathroom drifting with the aromas of scented candles and essential oils, a warm bright sunroom with its own daybed and crisp, fresh white linen, a reclining chair in a quiet forgotten corner surrounded by books and written wisdoms, or an artist's retreat alive with colour and creativity, strewn with canvas and paints.

Whatever and wherever your own special place is, the important thing is that you have one, that you recognise that you deserve one and that when you do have a few minutes of spare time you will make the effort to retreat to your oasis, recharge your batteries and soothe your soul.

To make 'special time out' accessible, follow these tips:

- Choose a place that feels soothing and special to you even before you do anything to it.
- Think about what really relaxes you and makes you feel calm, serene and connected. This should be reflected in your special place in some way.

- Preserve your special place. Don't try to establish it in a corner of a frequented room that family members, babies and children will have access to. It should be out of the way and in a protected area to prevent it from becoming untidy, damaged or frequented by other people.

- Envision calm if you're decorating your space. Opt for calming colours, gentle, graceful decor, inviting scents and comfortable, aesthetically pleasing furniture.

- Don't make your special place high maintenance. We already have so much to do in our day-to-day lives and it can be difficult to even find that little bit of time to yourself – don't waste it cleaning and arranging.

- Celebrate your own style. It can be as elaborate or as gloriously simple and basic as you want – after all, it is *your* special place!

- Enjoy it and use it whenever you can.

MOTIVATION, MODERATION AND DETERMINATION

Motivation is a key factor in reaching your goals. It drives you on, maintains your momentum, increases your expectations and enables you to expand as a person. Moderation allows you to pace this growth and development so that the gains become your new way of life. And steady progressive gains help sustain your determination to keep going.

The attributes needed to get motivated and stay motivated always reside within you – they include your inner drive, your inner beliefs, your inner ambitions.

When you believe in yourself, appreciate yourself and want the best for yourself, you will feel motivated to grow, to be the very best version of yourself that you can be. You will have the wisdom and patience you need to plan a progressively more challenging exercise program for yourself, and to develop a healthy sustainable relationship with food and eating.

Too many times I overdid it at the start of a new health regime or lifestyle change. I failed because I set myself such a gruelling, unrealistic exercise routine that my body would feel ripped and worn – after a few days or maybe a week I'd give up, feeling exhausted, depressed and defeated. How vividly I recall trying to follow a fast-paced expert-level fitness video or step class, or undertake a long run, only to feel humiliated by my disastrous attempt.

There were also times when I banished all carbs, fats, sugars and even healthy and necessary foods from my life as well as skipping meals. Then I would end up feeling starving, deprived, constipated and short tempered, lose a couple of kilos and put them straight back on when I returned to emotionally charged eating habits. Sometimes, I binged on unhealthy fattening foods because I was planning on starting a diet the next day. When I did try fad diets I found them too hard to follow, having to make separate meals for myself, spending extra money to achieve this, and feeling tired and hungry all the time.

Why is it that so many of us set ambitious lifestyle goals and new year's resolutions, start out with great enthusiasm and determination, yet flounder or give up entirely within a few days or weeks? Why is it that some women, on the other hand, are able to set themselves personal challenges and use them as catalysts for growth, experience and self improvement?

As one who had failed time and time again at countless diets and exercise routines, I had all but given up on myself in the realm of achieving personal goals of health and fitness.

It was sheer frustration and despair that forced me out of the house with my baby and the pram, to take that all-important life-changing walk. I returned home with a new appreciation of myself and faith in my capacity to take charge of my own wellbeing. From that momentous turning point, my self esteem improved and strengthened and I learned to appreciate not only myself but the many positives in my life.

I started focusing on what I valued, both in myself and in my situation, and found the following attitudes supportive and motivational:

- Appreciate and value your willingness to make healthy changes and take better care of yourself.
- Start focusing on what is right in your life and stop focusing on negatives.
- Stop focusing on what you are not, and instead focus on who you are and who you know you can become.

- Appreciate how fortunate you are (this might include appreciation for a beautiful child or partner, for the blessing of being a mother, for your home).
- Appreciate the pluses of where you live.
- Appreciate that right now you have a perfect opportunity to prove to yourself that you can become a healthy, energetic and confident version of yourself.
- Appreciate the opportunity to become a great role model for your child and for others.
- Appreciate that becoming healthy and active can actually be fun and exciting.

Remember it has taken years of learned behaviours and habits to become who you are right now. By appreciating the positive aspects of your existing self, and moving towards beneficial change one achievable step at a time, you are actually teaching yourself a sustainable new way of being and living.

When you start with achievable targets and work your way up each rung of the ladder to your ultimate goal the challenges no longer seem overwhelming. Taking the time to understand and appreciate all the milestones and successes along the way is so uplifting and exciting that you want to keep going. You stay motivated, you enjoy the journey and you succeed.

The more you achieve, the more you know you can achieve and the more motivated you become. Achieving self-improvement goals generates and sustains positive, healthy personal growth.

Whether you have set out to become more active, to lose weight, to eat more healthily, to ease depression or to de-clutter your life, the best and surest way of achieving success is by building the momentum one positive step at a time. It only takes that one small step, just a few small changes and the motivation will flow.

Motherhood

When you become happy with yourself and within yourself you are better able to fully appreciate the miracle and blessing that is motherhood. By dropping unrealistic expectations, needless worry over things you cannot change and taking the time to appreciate yourself you can savour more moments, enjoy more days and find pleasure in the little things. You come to realise that the key to being a wonderful mother is not age, background, income, experience, or situation. It is love – love of your child, love of your family, love of life, love of yourself.

Becoming a mother is the best thing that ever happened to me. It has forced me to grow. It has given me a new respect for and perception of the world around me. And it has caused me to rejoice in the small things and let go of negativity. The purity, honesty, trust, love and exciting possibilities that radiate from a new child generate a positive energy that encompasses the mother as well. My daughter inspires me to be true to myself and believe in myself. She inspires me to be all that I can be and to be the very best version of myself. I had never felt so strong and so capable, so fulfilled and confident. Being a mother has challenged me to learn new ways of being and thinking and to master the many skills that come with parenthood. It has motivated me to live more healthily and to feel good about myself.

Being a mother brings to my life an essence of pure joy.

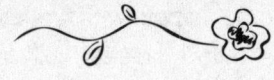

The Pram Diet Lifestyle

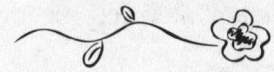

The basic principles that underpin the pram diet philosophy can be summarised in a page or two. Here they are:

- **Become an active, healthy person.**
- **Use what is already at your disposal** as your exercise equipment – namely, your pram and good old-fashioned walking in the fresh air.
- **Be a positive role model** for your children by improving your own lifestyle.
- **Learn to appreciate and be kind to yourself.**
- **Develop the motivational tools** you need to inspire you to successful weight loss that you can easily maintain.
- **Eat a healthy, balanced diet** that includes whole

grains, fresh fruits and vegetables, and quality protein. Use simple recipes that taste great and can be enjoyed by the whole family (see the menu and recipe section starting on page 148).

- **Become more involved with the foods you consume.** Learn about nutrition, and form a healthy relationship with food.
- **Grow some of your own veggies.** Eating foods you have grown yourself is beneficial in so many ways, for you and for your children. (There is an entire section devoted to this, starting on page 97.)
- **Discover where to shop economically for the freshest ingredients** – meat, seafood, poultry, fruits, vegetables and herbs.
- **Reward yourself** with non-food-based treats.
- **Find a creative outlet** and spend regular time being creative.
- **Designate and nurture a special place** that is your oasis in a hectic home environment.
- **Enjoy your progress.** Losing weight and improving your lifestyle should not be considered a quick fix but rather a steady-paced long-term program giving achievable results that you can easily maintain for the rest of your life.
- **Build a community.** Form or join support and friendship groups where you can exercise and socialise with other mothers. Encourage the children to interact with each other in active ways, and become fit and healthy mums together.

Once you have made the decision to change your life for the better you will find you feel a little lighter. You will begin to realise the personal power you possess – to understand how much control you can really have over your health, wellbeing and happiness.

Even so, there may be times when old unhelpful habits threaten to creep back in. At times like these, I found 'moving mantras' incredibly helpful. Chanting a mantra as you go about your daily chores or when you're out walking can be like having your very own cheer squad. A mantra is your personal cheer that encourages you to keep looking forward, to stay focused on your goals. It can give you a much-needed boost when things get tough.

Here are the mantras I used to cheer me on:

- **'I can and I am.'** I can and I am, I can and I am, I can and I am, I can and I am, I can and I am, I can and I am. This one is fantastic for pushing yourself that little bit further, keeping the motivation flowing, helping you to believe in yourself. It reminds you that you are already on the path to a better you and that you *are* already doing great things, *will* keep going and really *can* do it!

- **'I'd rather feel fabulous than eat lots of bad foods.'** I would repeat this whenever I found myself thinking of returning to old food triggers or bad habits (and this can happen, because we are human and we have spent a lot of time creating the bad habits in the first place; it takes time and perseverance to unlearn them completely). This mantra kept me focused on eating the fresh healthy foods that make you feel alive, full of energy, vibrant and looking wonderful.

- **'Just keep moving.'** Whether you are gathering momentum for a long walk, doing exercises, completing a set of weights, running errands by walking around town, or finding creative ways to be active around the house, you can maintain an energetic rhythm by repeating this mantra: 'Just keep moving, just keep moving, just keep moving, just keep moving, just keep moving.'
- **'Just a little bit more.'** A great mantra to help you build staying power, to keep you going when you feel like giving up.
- **'It's my life and now I'm really living it.'** Taking responsibility for your own life immediately helps you feel empowered. A sense of self empowerment generates motivation, helps you access the inner drive to become the best version of yourself. It supports you in following your dreams, focusing on how you want your life to be, finding what makes you happy and healthy, and filling your life with that.
- **'Day by day, in some way, I am improving.'** An excellent daily mantra, especially on those days when everything seems routine and change is not immediately evident.
- **'I feel good and look good because now I live so well.'** A little self esteem booster to chant when

you're looking in the mirror. Chant it proudly when you have achieved a weight loss goal and are trying on a new outfit, or after you've genuinely accepted a compliment.

START YOUR DAY FRESH

Every day is special, and each new day holds the promise of endless opportunities and fresh starts. Regardless of how bad yesterday was, how bad your night's sleep might have been (especially if you have a wakeful little one, or are deep in the throes of night feeds, teething, or illness), you can teach yourself to follow these simple steps that give your day a fresh, calm and energised start full of potential and zing.

- **Wake slowly.** Upon waking, no matter what chaos may be going on around you, take the time to stretch out fully on your bed. Stretch until you actually feel longer. Wriggle your toes and fingers, really feel every joint, every muscle, every part of your body getting ready for the new day. Rotate each of your ankles in three slow circles and open and close your hands a few times, loosening up your whole body.

- **Relax your mind.** Close your eyes for a moment and take three deep, slow breaths while picturing a place of pure serenity and peace – a beautiful beach on a glorious sunny day with warm sand and cool tranquil waters; a magical ancient forest filled with the sounds of rustling foliage and the calls of rare birds; a field of fragrant flowers radiant in the early morning sun; a gentle flowing creek hidden in the woods, alive with frogs and edged with delicate ferns and flowers. Whatever it is you envision, really feel yourself there – feel the sand between your toes, feel awe in the presence of those giant, mighty trees, feel that warming sun and smell those flowers, hear the soothing sounds of the water burbling in the creek. Take a minute or two to immerse yourself in serenity, and relax your mind.

- **Love today.** Open your eyes slowly and with confidence, and in a strong voice say the following words, 'I love today!' Then smile – smile like there is never going to be a reason not to, smile like you have not a care in the world, smile because you are so worth it, smile because it is a new day.

- **Gently wash your face** with fresh cool water before looking at your gorgeous self in the mirror and saying, 'I am a beautiful and amazing woman who is getting fitter and healthier and feeling better about myself each and every day. I do truly love being me'. Then give yourself a big genuine smile!

- **Start your day with a healthy energy-boosting breakfast.** Refer to the section on daily meal planners and recipes for tasty ideas (starting on page 132). Follow the healthy eating plan and read the suggestions to get you motivated to eat well in the morning. (Because you have used the shopping list suggestions, your home will already be filled with real foods and delicious fresh ingredients.)

- **Make your bed.** This is one bit of housework you really shouldn't let slide – it symbolically separates night from day, reinforcing the fresh start every morning.

- **Change out of your pyjamas.** Even if you are a stay-at-home mum or work from home, by getting dressed into fresh clothes soon after waking you will feel more awake and ready for a new day. Try to have some comfortable and fun clothes or outfits for those days at home. Invest in some simple day clothes that make you feel attractive – some brightly coloured singlets, soft warm sweaters and cardigans, tailored tracksuit pants that are flattering, simple but cute summery dresses. Celebrate your own style.

- **Spend a little bit of time on your appearance.** It doesn't have to be dramatic – just a few minutes spent doing your hair and perhaps applying a little make-up so you feel pretty and fresh. Being a mum, feeling tired or depressed, spending the day at home with your little one, not going anywhere special, can all be excuses for not bothering with your appearance. Make sure you spend a little time on yourself, for yourself!

- **Freshen up your house.** Make sure there is a good flow of fresh air through your home to clean out all the stale air of yesterday. This is especially important if you use air conditioning or heating.

- **Push that pram!** If you're an at-home mum, leave the housework until later and go for an early morning walk. You will come back full of vitality and energy, and feeling virtuous because you have done some exercise early in the day. If work or other commitments make this difficult, make sure you create time in your afternoon for that all-important walk. Better still, get up that bit earlier each morning and walk – yes, you are worth the effort and yes, you will feel wonderful for it.

- **Cultivate positivity.** A bouncy, happy attitude doesn't come naturally to all of us, and sometimes life's events and situations make it all but impossible to feel truly happy. But feeling down, angry, frustrated and stressed really does nothing to change the situation. Dwelling on the negatives, getting upset over things we cannot change, just makes us and those around us feel even more miserable. No matter how tough life is, there are usually positives that you can choose to focus on.

PRAM THERAPY FOR BODY, MIND AND SOUL

Prams are amazing weight-loss tools! They really are. Have you ever pushed your pram up a steep hill, across a grass verge, through sand, or for a long distance? Then you'll know just how much effort this actually takes!

Once you embrace the pram diet, you will find yourself deliberately pushing your pram across all those grass verges and up all those hills. Here are some tips to help you gain the most from every walk:

- **Posture.** When you go pram walking, make sure your body is relaxed but as straight as possible, and use those stomach muscles with every step – really feel the effort in your stomach, and feel it becoming firmer with every push. Your leg, arm and back muscles will strengthen up as well.

- **Walk at baby's nap time.** With babies or toddlers it can be hard to get going. I always timed my pram walk to coincide with Lily's morning nap and packed her pram with supplies so I wouldn't have to worry about turning back. Even if I had to stop and breast feed to get her off to sleep, I was out of the house and doing something that made me feel great. Lily loved it too.

- **Start out gently and build up pace and distance as your stamina improves.** Start with short gentle walks, gradually increasing the distance and difficulty of terrain as you grow stronger and fitter. I recommend you start by walking around two average suburban blocks. Do this for about two weeks, or less if you feel ready. Then increase two of the walks to four blocks and so on, until at least three times a week you are doing about a 5 kilometre walk quite comfortably.

- **Go for a walk at least five days a week.** It doesn't have to be a marathon – just a good brisk walk. The key – and I cannot stress this enough – is to make it interesting and enjoyable.
- **Increase the load.** Once you've gained a little confidence and fitness, add extra resistance by filling up your pram with toys, snacks and drinks for the little one, a first aid kit, change of clothes, nappy and blanket – anything you think you or your baby just might need.
- **Go shopping.** If your pram has a large underneath compartment and is well balanced with strong handles (so that you're sure it won't tip over), take it shopping! Three or four green bags full of shopping will really add resistance and increase your pram pushing strength. Combine this with parking your car at the very back of the carpark and you will be surprised at how many calories you burn. Find a good safe carpark in the centre of an area where you plan to visit a few stores, run some errands or even get lunch. Pack up your pram and, using your car as base, walk to each of the different stores. Consider making a day or a morning of it – visit the library, eat lunch in a park, stop for a coffee.
- **Take your pram on adventures.** Walk in a national park, along a beach, a coastal cycleway, through a park. Walk to the shops, walk to a post box to post a letter, walk to a local shop and buy yourself the newspaper or a magazine, go for a picnic with

your little one, take them to the park, the beach, a friend's house. Walk whenever you can.

- **Walk with friends.** Take a friend with you for support and to motivate each other, or go for a picnic with another mum and her baby. Start a mums' walking group in your area or meet somewhere interesting and make it an exciting outing for mothers and babies alike.
- **Walk for fun.** Take your dog, your friend's dog or even your iPod. Whatever your style, just make sure it's fun!

The walk should be something you enjoy and look forward to each day. Eventually you might not even want to have two days off a week – you might want to walk 5 kilometres every day! The potential gains are phenomenal and the enjoyment you will receive from pram walking is truly endless. Always remember to make it fun and you will find that the walk can be the day's highlight for both you and your little one. Once your little one is older, you might even take up bushwalking, mountain climbing or become a professional dog walker.

By using your pram as your exercise tool of choice you will be developing an active routine that involves your child, making exercise a really positive lifestyle and bonding experience. As your child grows you can progress from the pram to a stroller and on to a parent push-trike before eventually advancing to walking alongside the child as they ride their bike.

Exercise produces feel-good endorphins, gets your blood circulating and gives you an overall sense of wellbeing. It benefits your mind and soul as much as it benefits your body. There will always be plenty of housework, but there is only one you. Sometimes you just have to give your own health and happiness top priority. Most families would rather come home to a happy, glowing mum and a few dishes in the sink than to an immaculate house and a stressed out, exhausted mother.

BEYOND THE PRAM – OTHER EXERCISE OPTIONS

It is so important to push your body into a sweat each and every day. By using your creativity and resourcefulness you will find there are so many daily chores and activities that can be turned into fun and exercise. Add these to your regular pram walking routine and you are on a fast track to a healthier, fitter and stronger you.

Even the simplest of tasks, when viewed from a different angle, can work different muscle groups, build strength and tone different parts of your body. There are so many ways we can get an unexpected workout around the home and in everyday life. Here are just a few ideas to get you thinking:

- vigorously mopping the floors
- enthusiastically washing the windows

- vacuuming the whole house thoroughly at a fast pace
- manually emptying the bath water onto the gardens after the kids have their bath, with a bucket
- digging in the veggie patch
- playing chasings with a toddler
- holding your posture straight and doing a slow, steady squat every time you pick up a toy or piece of clothing from the floor (you'll be surprised how many times you squat in the course of a day)
- giving your bathroom(s) a really good 'going over' with a scrubbing brush and scourer
- watering some of your gardens with a watering can, alternating the arm you use to build strength in each arm or using two watering cans and doing slow purposeful lifts and lowering movements as you walk along
- playing cricket with the kids
- using a shovel and wheelbarrow to spread a load of topsoil around your gardens
- spreading mulch over all your gardens
- walking the kids to school
- going for an afternoon bike ride with the whole family
- always parking at the very back of shopping centres, so you have further to walk

There are so many ways to get your heart rate up and your body burning calories – use your imagination and see what you discover. Even gently rocking a baby or toddler to sleep can give your arms a workout, as can commando crawling across the floor with your little one, sweeping a long driveway or dancing with your children.

Put your mind to it and you will be amazed at just how easy it is to get physical. You might even be able to convert some of the most dreaded chores into workouts.

Once your transformation really gets under way, you are bound to lose some weight. Whenever you lose weight, especially if it is a large amount, even though you feel fitter and trimmer you can be left with areas of your body that lack definition and toning. That is when some additional daily exercises can really come into their own. And remember – by toning and building muscle you will find it even easier to maintain a healthy weight for the rest of your life.

Here are a few simple exercises for toning and strength-building at home, but before you start, remember these important points:

- *Always have a checkup with your doctor before undertaking any new form of physical activity or exercise.*
- *Always begin with a small number of repetitions and work your way up gradually.*
- *Always stretch before and after any exercise.*
- *Being fit and healthy isn't just about looking good – it's about feeling good too.*

- **The mini push-up.** This exercise is also known as the lady push-up, the half push-up and the intermediate push-up. Get down on the floor on your hands and knees, arms straight. Your hands should be positioned slightly wider than your shoulders. Tighten your stomach muscles by pulling your navel up towards your spine – your body should look strong and straight, with a flat back. Without moving your legs, slowly lower your torso, bending at the elbows and keeping your back straight, then push up, and repeat. Be realistic to begin with – 10 repeats will be plenty. Gradually increase the number of repeats until you can comfortably do around 50 mini push-ups.

- **The furniture sit-up.** *Caution: it is very easy to do sit-ups incorrectly and cause injury to your neck or back.* Bracing your feet under something heavy like a piece of furniture forces you to use your stomach muscles to do all the work. All you need is an item of furniture like a bed, sofa or wardrobe that is sturdy and stable and that also has a gap underneath it where you can 'hook' your feet. Lie on your back on a mat, with your knees bent and your feet flat on the floor beneath the item of furniture. Cross your arms over your chest, with a hand on each shoulder. Your back, neck and shoulder muscles should be relaxed, and your back should remain straight. Using only your stomach muscles, lift your torso into a sitting position and then lower it gently back to

73

the mat. Check to make sure you are feeling the effort in your stomach and that all the lifting is coming from those muscles. Start with 10 repeats, gradually increasing the number of sit-ups to 50 as your stomach muscles become stronger.

- **The wall squat.** This exercise is excellent for working your thighs, including your inner thighs. Make sure you are wearing clothing that won't 'catch' or be damaged from rubbing against a wall. Stand straight with your back to a wall, legs shoulder width apart. Either cross your arms over your chest, place a hand on each hip or hold a small weight in each hand as you lower yourself into a squat, then raise yourself up again, always keeping your back flat against the wall. Start with 10 wall squats and progress to 50 as your thighs become stronger.

- **Touch your toes.** Stand up straight, feet a little further than shoulder width apart. Make sure both feet are pointed to the front and your stance is comfortable. Stretch your left arm up, then reach it over towards your right foot. Keep your legs straight, bend from the waist and relax your neck so that your head hangs loose. Using your stomach muscles and raising your left arm, return to the straight standing position. Repeat the exercise with your right arm stretching towards your left foot. Begin by reaching only as far as you comfortably can, aiming eventually to touch your toes. Alternate arms at a reasonable pace for best results, increasing the number of repetitions as you become stronger and more flexible. Be sure to keep your legs straight so that your stomach muscles and arms are doing most of the work.

- **The leg lift.** This is great for firming up your buttocks. Get down on your hands and knees, hands approximately shoulder width apart, back held strong and straight, stomach muscles tight. Lift one knee off the ground, then stretch that leg straight out behind you, holding the weight with the rest of your body. Hold that position for 10 seconds, then bend the knee and gently lower it back towards the floor, but do not put it down. Straighten and bend the same leg 10 times, then swap sides and repeat the exercise 10 times with the other leg.

- **The D.** Lie down flat on your back (you may want to lie on a mat), arms straight down beside your body and legs stretched out straight. Tighten your stomach muscles by pulling your navel in towards your spine. Raise your right leg only and lift it straight up to make a 45 degree angle with the floor, using your stomach muscles to keep the rest of your body firmly on the ground. Point the toes of your right foot and draw a large D shape in the air, using your whole leg (kept straight) in the movement. Draw 10 Ds before lowering your right leg gently to the ground. Repeat with your left leg, remembering that the D will be mirror image (straight side running in line with the centre of your body).

Gaining real muscle tone, fitness and strength leaves you feeling energised and healthy, makes your body work more efficiently and increases your body image confidence. It also opens up a whole new world of experiences and activities that may previously have appeared too daunting, difficult or just plain out of reach.

Being fitter and stronger often goes hand in hand with a more active and exciting lifestyle. There are so many activities you can try:

- Going to the gym (no longer a scary prospect when you feel confident that you are fit and strong).
- Signing up for a physical class such as water aerobics, self defence, surfing, ballroom dancing, abseiling, or rock climbing.
- Participating in a sport. Not only is organised sport a good way of keeping fit and being active, it is also a great way to meet friends and have fun.
- Seeing more of your world by bushwalking, mountain climbing, taking nature walks, exploring the great outdoors, going on adventure outings as a family.
- Being fit and active with your children – going for a long bike ride together, having a go at rollerblading with them at the local park, playing a game of beach volleyball or backyard cricket.
- Setting targets to work towards, such as walking 6 kilometres easily every day, participating in a marathon, being able to run a mile in a certain time frame or doing 10 laps of the public swimming pool on a regular basis.

A NEW RELATIONSHIP WITH FOOD

Along with walking and other physical exercise, the transformational journey to an increased sense of wellbeing, strong self esteem, good health and happiness involves clearing out all our old damaging habits and attitudes relating to foods, diets, nutrition and food preparation.

Since we spend most of our food preparation time in the kitchen, it's a great place to start building our new relationship with food.

Here, in more detail, are the foundations of the pram diet approach to foods, eating and food preparation:

- **Clean out your kitchen (literally).** Put aside a day or afternoon when you can devote some time to this (if you have a baby or toddler, ask a family member of friend to look after them for a while, so you are distraction free). Give the whole kitchen, including the pantry, cupboards, oven, fridge and freezer, a really thorough clean. Pick a day just before you're due to do your regular food shopping so you that can restock your fridge and cupboards in their newly clean, fresh state. Discard all foods that are past their use-by date, contain lots of artificial ingredients, are high in sugar, salt, fats or preservatives, or are excessively processed. Reorganise your storage system by investing in stackable airtight plastic containers to keep your foods fresh while making more kitchen space available. Introduce a labelling system on the containers and store them in a practical, organised way so that it's easy for all the family to find what they're looking for. Cane baskets and attractive bowls or boxes are another great way to store and display foods that do not need to be kept airtight in your cupboards. Spend serious time on the storage and display of your foods – be creative and make the system appealing and user friendly. Once your pantry and kitchen are clean, fresh and organised it's time to go shopping. Follow the shopping list guide (see pages 87–93) and locate the best source of fresh fruit and vegetables in your area.

- **Eat regularly.** In particular, do not skip breakfast (see pages 148–155 for some great appetising breakfast ideas). It is vital to eat breakfast and to eat regularly to keep your metabolism firing, burning calories and to maintain energy levels so you are ready to take on a full and exciting day. (Yes, even being an at-home mum with a Mount Everest-sized pile of washing and an arm-long list of chores can be exciting, if you let it be by being a bit creative.) Eating three main meals, plus two to three healthy snacks, or six small meals per day, you keep your body and metabolism evenly fuelled and help to reduce overeating and binge eating. Eat smaller portions at every meal and eat when you are sitting down and conscious of the act. Never eat on the run, pick at food while running about the house or nibble in front of the TV. If you do, you will have no real concept of how much you have eaten, nor will you really appreciate the meal.

- **Eat slowly!** This is so important. Eating too fast can lead to constipation, bowel problems, indigestion, and weight gain from eating past the full stage.

- **Eat nutritious, healthy snacks and meals** made from deliciously fresh ingredients (see pages 132 and 148 for daily meal planner ideas and recipes).

- **Prepare yourself healthy snacks and nibbles.** Set up some containers in your fridge, car and pantry that you can easily access when you feel like snacking. One should contain pieces of fresh chopped up fruits like watermelon and rockmelon, whole strawberries and blueberries; others should contain more savoury treats like different types of seeds, plain, unsalted popcorn, raw walnuts and rice crackers.

- **Drink plenty of water.** Being properly hydrated is the key to an efficient and healthy body. If you find your local tap water not very appealing, try using a water filtration system or purchasing a water filter jug. Alternatively, you could look at installing a rain water tank. Remember, the more active you are the more you should drink to rehydrate yourself. Invest in a permanent water bottle that you can take everywhere with you in the car, to the shops, to work, on an outing, when visiting friends and so on. Drink a big glass of water whenever you feel a sugar or snack craving. A little trick is to teach yourself your own personal mantra that you can repeat in moments of temptation or frustration; something like: 'drink more water, drink more water, drink more water'. Don't wait until you are thirsty to have a drink – when you feel thirsty you are already slightly dehydrated. And remember, dehydration can lead to fluid retention, feeling lethargic, bad skin and many other health problems. Water is a beautiful revitalising liquid that is an essential part of a healthy and happy body and is required by each and every human being. Yet somewhere along the way, most of us have lost the ability to appreciate, savour and enjoy the taste and sensation of a glass of cool fresh water.

- **Schedule a cooking day.** This is a day, or a few hours at night, in the morning or during an afternoon that you set aside once a week or fortnight to make up some healthy meals and freeze them. Then, on those nights when you are just too tired, unwell, really busy, want to give yourself some pampering, are occupied with your children, just want to relax, or would rather go for a walk, you can pop a ready-made meal in the oven and let dinner prepare itself.

- **Grow some of your own** lovely fruit, vegetables and herbs. This is especially good if you have children – they will love it, and you will be teaching them skills, valuable knowledge and a healthy understanding and appreciation of food. Trust me – you will have no problem getting kids to eat veggies they've grown and nurtured themselves, and you've turned into a delicious dish. Children are a huge help in looking after a veggie patch and if you don't have children or they're too young, do it for yourself! Not only is gardening therapeutic and good exercise – it is also very rewarding. You save money and gain a real feeling of accomplishment and pride when you harvest your very own organic fresh ingredients (see pages 97–130 for details on how to establish and maintain your own food garden). Nothing tastes quite as good as home-grown.

REAL FOODS AND REAL WEIGHT LOSS

It is important when starting the pram diet to remember that it is a complete life makeover and not a 'quick fix' diet that is difficult to maintain and generally ineffective in the long run. With the pram diet, you are starting your life afresh, with new respect for food and yourself.

No food should ever be considered a luxury item or forbidden – that just creates negative associations. On the pram diet, you can still have a piece of chocolate cake, a glass of red wine or a slice of pizza occasionally because you are learning to understand and appreciate foods better and you know what your body needs to function well.

In any case, by eating a proper balanced diet with plenty of whole foods, whole grains, good quality protein, fresh fruits and vegetables, you will feel less inclined to overindulge on high calorie foods. When you routinely eat regular healthy meals and snacks, and drink lots of water, the cravings for greasy and salty foods or a 'sugar hit' will fade away.

By planning your day, including your personal menu, you can factor in a chocolate biscuit with your afternoon cup of coffee, or a toasted cheese and bacon sandwich on that lunch date. Just balance out the extra calories by adjusting the other foods you eat in that day, and making sure you get plenty of exercise. Here's another example: by eating a healthy fruit and yogurt breakfast, fresh salad with low-fat dressing for lunch and steamed vegetables and tofu with brown rice for dinner, you can allow a glass of red wine with your meal plus a few squares of a rich dark chocolate for dessert that night – consume them slowly and really enjoy them. It's important that you do not view the biscuit, wine and chocolate as treats or rewards – rather, include them as occasional menu items.

Foods to include in your healthy eating plan

The following foods and ingredients are all excellent for those trying to lose excess weight or simply eat more healthily. They are either low in calories and fat, really healthy for you or are great at getting your metabolism going.

- **High fibre foods** are so good for you in so many ways. They clean you out, speed up your metabolism, leave you feeling fuller longer, are an excellent source of energy and keep your whole system working more efficiently and burning calories. Even when you are sleeping! They include: whole grains and whole grain products, fresh fruit and vegetables (particularly raw), lentils, pulses and dried fruit.

- **Fresh foods in season.** Almost any food in its fresh or natural state is fantastic for your wellbeing and health. Think juicy oranges, chunks of watermelon, a ripe red tomato, fresh-picked strawberries, a celery stick from the garden, a handful of crisp fresh runner beans.

- **Heart friends.** Yes, there are foods that are great for your heart! And a healthy and happy heart is important for a healthy and happy body. These include: avocado, walnuts, hazelnuts, almonds, salmon and other oily fish, blueberries, flaxseed oil, spinach, pears, good quality cold pressed olive oil.

- **High quality low-fat protein.** Protein is critical for maintaining muscle health and strength, in fact, good health in general. At least 10 per cent and up to a third of your daily food intake should be protein. The best sources are legumes (like peas, beans and lentils), poultry, eggs, seafood, lean red meat, dairy products, nuts and seeds.

- **Hot and spicy foods.** Generally, 'what heats you up speeds you up', meaning that hot and spicy foods can kick-start your metabolism into working at a slightly faster pace. Consider ingredients like:

chilli, pepper, wasabi, curry and hot spices and herbs.

- **Herbs and spices** are so versatile. They can add tantalising flavours to your cooking, removing the need for added salt, sugar and fats. Many are aromatic, have practical uses around the home, or are invaluable companion plants in your gardens and veggie patch. Some herbs are valued for their therapeutic or healing qualities. A few basics: parsley, basil, oregano, thyme, bay leaves, allspice, paprika, cinnamon, nutmeg, cumin, coriander.

Foods to limit and avoid

The following foods are either really high in calories and fats or are unhealthy for other reasons. Foods I included in this list are best avoided, or consumed in very limited quantities, occasionally.

- **White bread, white flour, white rice and pasta.** Not only are they usually bleached and chemically treated, they are also stripped of most of their fibre and goodness. Do not be fooled by sneaky advertising – go for the whole grains every time! Choose healthy options like brown rice, wild rice, wholemeal flour, whole grain breads, whole grain pasta, wholemeal crackers and whole grain breakfast cereals.
- **Salty foods.** Too much salt can be really bad for your health and can lead to bloating and water

retention. Many processed and pre-packaged foods (including quite a few you wouldn't think of) are very high in salt, so it is always important to read the labels on food packaging (see page 87). Substitute herbs and spices for salt in your cooking whenever you can, and resist the urge to sprinkle salt on your food.

- **Full fat dairy products,** including yellow cheese, cream, yogurt, ice cream, sour cream, milk, milk chocolate and white chocolate.

- **Pastry goods,** including croissants, fruit pies, meat pies and sausage rolls, store-bought quiche. Most pastry is made with margarine or butter and contains lots of hidden calories.

- **Deep-fried foods.** Look for healthier options when buying takeaway. Consider options like sushi, salad wraps in wholemeal breads without the creamy sauces, a freshly made salad sandwich minus the butter and mayonnaise, fruit salad, a low-fat burger, grilled chicken and salad, or steamed fish with vegetables. At home, swap the deep-fried chips for oven-baked wedges of sweet potato, carrot and pumpkin with garlic and herbs.

- **Takeaway and processed foods.** They are generally high in calories and low in fibre and nutritional benefits. If you are buying prepared food, see the previous list for relatively healthy suggestions.

- **Sugary foods.** Not only are they very high in calories and damaging to your teeth – they also increase your risk of developing diabetes and other illnesses.

- **Potatoes** are not bad for you but when you are trying to lose weight they can hinder your progress, simply because they are high-energy carbohydrates. Don't cut potatoes out altogether, but do reduce the amount you consume and try steaming or boiling instead or roasting them. Where possible, replace them with sweet potato or pumpkin.

HEALTHY FOOD SHOPPING

There are so many food shopping options available to us as consumers in our society – well-stocked supermarkets, greengrocers, butchers and seafood vendors, community and farmers' markets, health food stores and bulk food wholesalers. Collectively they offer a vast selection of healthy foods, flavourings and pre-packaged meals. With so many choices available, choosing only nutritious healthy foods and ingredients can seem daunting at first.

First, familiarise yourself with the foods and food groups discussed on pages 82–84. Then go through your kitchen and your healthy recipe collection (see pages 132–207, and make a master list of every food and ingredient you would like to stock in your cupboards, fridge and freezer. Whenever you plan to go food shopping, refer to this master list, and write a shopping list of everything you need to buy. Finally, familiarise yourself with the labelling systems used on packaged foods – being able to read and understand the labels will increase your confidence and make it simpler for you to choose healthy foods.

***

Reading food labels

Australia has strict laws governing what must be listed on the labels of manufactured and packaged foods. Remember, the ingredients are listed in order according to what proportion of the product they make up. The law also requires the nutritional breakdown of the product to be listed, showing how much fat, sugar, salt, carbohydrate and protein it contains, proportionally. Just because something is advertised as 'fat free' or 'low in fat' doesn't always mean it is healthy or low in calories – it could be full of sugar and/or salt. Items like lollies and soft drinks, for example, might contain no fat at all, but have extremely high sugar (and therefore calorie) content. Foods high in all or any of these (fat, sugar and salt) are not in your best interests.

***

The shopping list

This is the master list from which I write my weekly shopping list. It contains foods, food types, varieties, flavourings, condiments and beverages that fit well into the pram diet and successful and maintainable weight loss. They are foods that either have health benefits, are nutritious and filling, are low in fat, calories and sugar or are wholesome and nurturing to both the mind and the body.

Fruit, so full of natural goodness, fibre and vitamins. Keep plenty of different varieties on hand at all times. Buy what's in season and be sure to check out local fresh fruit markets, farm gate stalls and farmers' markets as well as your local supermarket.

Vegetables. Keep one shelf and the crisper drawers in your fridge full of fresh vegetables. This will ensure that you always have the makings of healthy and delicious meals. Using lots of fresh vegetables in your cooking and snacks will provide you and your family with much of the nutrition and fibre you need to maintain good health. If you don't grow a lot of your vegetables or source them from a local market, they should be taking up a large proportion of your shopping trolley. Plan your weekly menu in advance to ensure every meal includes fresh vegetables. Buy what's in season, taking advantage of specials and bulk purchases – you can save money and will be inspired to explore less familiar vegetables.

Herbs and spices are essential for flavouring healthy meals and reducing the need for excess salt, sugar and fats. Buy spices in small quantities and store them, clearly labelled, in airtight containers; they are best used within a few weeks or months of being packaged. If possible, buy spices whole and grind small quantities as you need them.

There are many different herbs offering a wide variety of flavours and functions. As some are toxic or dangerous, it's a good idea to learn a bit about herbs before you start using them in your cooking. Also, a good herb combination can make a meal taste fantastic, but a bad herb combination can ruin a meal. Do some research on herbs – have a chat to qualified nursery staff, any chefs you know, and experienced gardeners. Borrow books from your local library and decide what herbs might suit you and your tastes. Grow selected herbs in your garden, so they will be beautifully fresh and full of flavour.

Herbs and spices are a big part of the secret to creating delicious healthy meals, so it's worth putting in the time and effort to learn about the ones that suit you and your family's tastes.

The following are great to use in many dishes and are generally easy to acquire and use: parsley, rosemary, thyme, mint, basil, lemon thyme, sage, chives, oregano, bay leaves, coriander, cinnamon, paprika, chilli, cumin, nutmeg, curry powders and pepper.

Other basics. Vegetable oils are excellent in salads and, consumed in moderation, can help reduce cholesterol levels. Cold pressed virgin oils are healthiest, as cold pressing does not destroy valuable nutrient content. You can find a wide range of oils in most supermarkets – some are excellent to use when stir-frying; others add a delicious flavour to salad dressings. Look for virgin olive oil, rice oil, avocado oil, mustard seed oil, linseed oil and flaxseed oil.

Free range eggs should be a staple in your pantry or fridge (depending on how warm the weather is). Free range (organic, if possible) are far superior in flavour, colour, texture and for cooking, and you are also supporting the farmers who treat their animals with respect and dignity.

Condiments, flavourings and sauces. Not everyone is partial to the taste of 'nude' foods. Children in particular sometimes resist unadorned fruit and vegetables. Often, adding a small amount of healthy dressing, sauce or other flavouring agent can transform the ordinary into the extraordinary. Try additions like dried herbs, stock cubes, dehydrated onion, sea salt (in small amounts), tomato relish, cocoa, peri peri sauce, soy sauce, oyster sauce, garlic, ginger, gravy powder, mustards, low-fat mayonnaise, fat-free salad dressings, tomato paste, light sweet and sour sauce, salsa, tomato-based pasta sauces, carob, coconut, light coconut milk and good quality vinegars. Be sure to check the labels of these products before you buy.

Cold foods. Keep your fridge well stocked with staples like low-fat cheeses (feta, ricotta, cream cheese, cottage cheese), low-fat and natural yogurt, low-fat milk, soy milk, real butter (to be used sparingly), low-fat sour cream, low-fat dips, hummus, tabouleh, tofu, low-fat ham, smoked salmon slices, vegetarian soy rashers, sausages, roasts and soya slices, low-fat meat cuts, skinless chicken pieces, fresh sustainably caught–grown fish, low-fat mince and Chinese noodles.

Frozen foods are great stand-by ingredients.

Keep your freezer well stocked with frozen foods like berries, low-fat pastry sheets (preferably whole grain), light fish fillets and uncoated fish fillets (bearing the sustainable fishing logo), shredded spinach, light ice cream or frozen yogurt, unbattered squid rings, skinless chicken and whole grain low-fat prepared meals.

Canned foods often save you time, while augmenting fresh fruits and vegetables in your meals. Choose organic where possible and keep a good store of them on hand in your pantry or cupboards. Include brown lentils, red kidney beans, borlotti beans, three bean mix, mexi beans, cannellini beans, refried beans, tuna in spring water, corn kernels, creamed corn, crushed or chopped tomatoes, whole peeled tomatoes, baked beans, asparagus, beetroot slices, peas, pineapple pieces and other fruits in natural juice, vegetarian 'meat' substitutes, chick peas, oysters in tomato sauce, tinned salmon (in brine or water), low-fat soups, low-fat curry sauce, Asian vegetables, bamboo shoots and artichokes.

Packet foods. Have a good look around the supermarkets, delicatessens and smaller stores in your area as there are many packaged whole grain and/or organic products now available – different stores often carry particular brands or offer different products. Packet foods to include in your shopping list are: whole grain lasagne sheets, pasta, cracker biscuits and crisp breads, cereals; wholemeal pasta, self raising flour, plain flour; rice, corn, soy or spelt pasta; taco shells, wild rice, brown rice, rice crackers, popcorn (natural or fat-free if pre-cooked), light low-fat crackers, falafel mix, couscous, ground flaxseeds, wheat germ, barley, dried lentils, dehydrated beans, chick peas, split peas, soup mix, low-fat muesli, rolled oat porridge, phylum husks, LSA mix or women's nutrient formula (usually found in the health food section of the supermarket or at a health food shop), and low-fat and low-sugar fruit bars and biscuits.

Treats and snack foods. Keep a supply of these in the cupboard and you will be much less tempted to revert to unhealthy snacking habits. Consider including: dark chocolate (preferably organic, at least 70 percent cocoa content), dried unsweetened fruit pieces, liquorice, sunflower seeds, sesame seeds, pepitas (pumpkin seeds), raw and unsalted walnuts, hazelnuts and almonds.

Beverages. Water is and always will be the very best thing you can drink. It's a good idea to install a rain water tank and a water filtration system, and buy a water filter jug for your fridge so that your home always has plenty of fresh, sweet tasting water available. Buy yourself and each of your family members a good quality personal water bottle and always fill it up before you leave the house, eliminating the inclination to be constantly buying refreshments. For those times when you want something a little different, try mineral water, soda water, low-fat soy milk, low-fat dairy milk, rice milk, herbal teas, organic white tea, organic fair trade coffee and organic black tea (limited to three cups per day), freshly squeezed vegetable juices and freshly made smoothies. If you drink alcohol, choose red wine, low carbohydrate beer like pure blonde or super dry, vodka with tomato juice or scotch on ice. Limit yourself to one standard drink, and only drink alcohol occasionally.

HEALTHY FOOD FOR SPECIAL OCCASIONS

Holidays and special occasions are times when family and friends get together, socialising, celebrating, relaxing and eating. It can be all too easy at such times to overindulge and eat large quantities of unhealthy foods or consume too much calorie-laden alcohol. Being a healthy, active, energised person can slip to the back of your mind or be put on hold until later.

But if you let this happen, how will you feel afterwards? How much of your hard work will be undone? How much more difficult will it be to reach your goal of being a slimmer, happier, healthier you? Would you actually enjoy yourself more if you were feeling really confident about yourself, and healthier at your ideal weight? Does the short-lived enjoyment of indulging in the typical high-calorie foods of the festive season leave you feeling bloated, guilty, unhappy and sluggish?

Well, the good news is that on the pram diet you *can* still have a fantastic time, eat really delicious foods and have lots of fun. By staying in control of what you consume and by thinking outside the square – for example, by offering to host the family get-together or party – you can ensure there are plenty of delicious, healthy foods on hand. If you are going to someone else's place for a dinner party or barbecue, take a plate of healthy food to share, or a platter of healthy nibbles and some delicious fresh fruit. That way, you can join in with the celebrations knowing that you're going to feel great afterwards.

When entertaining at home, or catering for large gatherings, there are some fabulous foods and serving suggestions that will guarantee you and your guests feel as though you're being treated like kings and queens.

Always serve plenty of fresh fruit. Fresh fruit is such an easy and attractive solution to providing healthy, appealing and delicious finger food for yourself, your guests and your family. There are so many varieties and flavours to choose from and fruit can be easily arranged to create stunning, stylish table centrepieces. For dessert, a fruit platter, fruit smoothies or freshly made fruit salad drizzled with passionfruit and topped with a low-fat custard or yogurt are all excellent options.

Prepare platters of healthy, tasty nibbles. Create interesting platters that guests can 'graze' on. Try some of these ideas:

- **Seafood twist** with cooked prawns, avocado pieces, cherry tomatoes, slices (approximately 1 centimetre thick) of cooked 'light' crumbed fish portions, fresh oysters, smoked salmon slices, raw red onion rings, fresh soft lettuce leaves, baby spinach leaves, carrot sticks, celery sticks, red capsicum slivers, fresh curly parsley sprigs. On the side, serve low-fat mayonnaise and low-fat thousand island dressing (or your own healthy homemade dressings) in small dipping bowls.

- **Crunchy dry platter** with rice crackers, unsalted and unbuttered natural popcorn, pretzels, raw unsalted walnuts, raw unsalted almonds, nuts in the shell, sunflower seeds, pepitas and microwaved pappadums.

- **Savoury platter** with hummus, low-fat dips, cubes of different low-fat cheeses, olives, semi sun-dried tomatoes (not in oil), water crackers, low-fat crispbreads, rice crackers, slices of red capsicum, slices of avocado, fat-free ham, slices of cucumber, cherry tomatoes or wedges of a firm ripe tomato, carrot sticks, celery sticks, parsley sprigs and hard-boiled eggs cut into quarters.

- **Sweet platter** with squares of a rich dark chocolate, cherries, grapes, apple wedges (a splash of fresh lemon juice will prevent them from turning brown), sultanas, dried apricots, dried figs, dried apple rings, prunes and dates. (A side dish with almonds and cubes of low-fat cheese complements this platter beautifully.)

- **Chicken platter** with pieces of grilled chicken (skin removed), slices of avocado, raw green beans, snow peas, slices of a low-fat cheese, homemade croutons, cherry tomatoes, cucumber, fresh pine-apple, plus boiled baby potatoes flavoured with mixed herbs, sea salt and cracked black pepper.

- **Fruit platter** with watermelon, rockmelon, honeydew melon, grapes, cherries, mango, paw paw, pineapple, banana, mandarin, orange, apple, blueberries, kiwifruit and figs.

Make great salads. Salads are popular at any gathering, dinner party or barbecue – the trick is to make them interesting and use really fresh ingredients. A tasty dressing is a must for a tantalising salad along with a good combination of flavours from fresh ingredients. Create healthy versions of old standards like potato salad dressed with low-fat mayonnaise, mustard, fresh chives and spring onions; healthy coleslaw with crisp cabbage, shredded carrot, finely-shredded beetroot, finely sliced onion, a sprinkling of tasty seeds and a zesty low-fat dressing; lush green salads bursting with a wide variety of flavours, colours and textures. Or turn to the recipe section starting on page 148 for more unusual salad ideas.

Develop a signature dish. Create and perfect a healthy dish that is your specialty, and people will look forward to eating at your place just to savour that dish. Here are a few ideas to get you thinking:

- **Homemade oven-roasted wedges** of sweet potato, pumpkin and carrot seasoned with fresh herbs and spices.

- **Steamed fresh fish and vegetables** with your own special homemade honey, herb and mustard or sweet chilli dressing.
- **Grilled Turkish bread.** Top the bread with organic tomato paste, low-fat cheese, garlic, baby spinach leaves and herbs. Grill it, then cut into small squares to serve.
- **Whole grain pasta bake** with lots of freshly chopped tomatoes, basil, parsley and chilli, topped with a sprinkling of low-fat cheese.
- **Pumpkin soup** made with your own homegrown delicious pumpkins and lots of fresh herbs.
- **Vegetable lasagne** with whole grain lasagne sheets, lots of fresh vegetables and low-fat ricotta cheese.

There really are so many healthy, tasty foods that you can serve. With a bit of planning, preparation, experimentation and imagination you can enjoy great foods on every occasion without feeling guilty, worrying about the sort of role model you might be or how much weight you will gain.

GROWING YOUR OWN FOOD

Eating delicious meals made from fresh ingredients is one of the things that makes living a healthy lifestyle such an enjoyable, rewarding experience. The best chefs in the world will tell you – the meal is nothing without quality ingredients. With a good supply of tasty, fresh, nutritious produce and easy, appetising recipes you are well equipped to succeed in your quest for a healthy diet. And as organic fruits and vegetables can be expensive or hard to find, I strongly recommend you consider growing at least some of your own!

Sourcing fresh, organically grown ingredients, especially when you're on a budget, is not always an easy undertaking. You might need to do a bit of sleuthing in your local area and on the internet. Remember, local fruit and vegetable markets are usually cheaper than most supermarkets, and the produce is generally fresher. It is often grown locally, which means it hasn't been transported long distances or stored for long periods of time.

Organic fruit and vegetables can often be found at local markets, health food stores and even some supermarkets, as many are branching into these lines. If your local supermarket doesn't stock organic produce at the moment don't be afraid to ask them to – after all, they want to keep their customers happy and usually appreciate feedback. It really is worth the extra money for fresh organic produce. It tastes fantastic and usually keeps fresher longer, making it better value in the long run. You are not consuming or feeding potentially harmful chemicals to your family. And you have the satisfaction of knowing you are supporting environmentally friendly food producers.

Even if you are a busy person, work long hours,

have a large family to look after, are worried about water restrictions, live in a small flat with only a tiny balcony, or have no gardening experience, you can still grow some sort of fresh produce for yourself and your family.

You could even get together with your neighbours, local school, church or community group and start a communal vegetable patch. Turn it into an educational experience for the children, and sell your excess organic produce to raise funds for seeds and equipment. This is a wonderful way to make friends, enjoy the outdoors and generate community bonding in your area.

Growing fruit and vegetables organically is fun. When you have an organic vegetable garden you will be rewarded, not only with an abundance of healthy food, but also with a fascinating array of photogenic 'wildlife' – worms, insects, slaters and birds, to name a few. Children of all ages find the garden ecosystem really interesting – and being involved in growing their own food is a fantastic, hands-on approach to learning.

You will feel a deep sense of pride and accomplishment when you harvest and eat your delicious home-grown produce and – trust me – you will have no trouble persuading children to eat vegetables they grew themselves, especially if you also involve them in the food preparation and cooking. Children who work in their own veggie patch develop solid foundations for a healthy lifestyle as well as understanding more about the food they consume, and where it comes from.

Getting down and dirty

Getting started can sometimes seem a daunting task. Veggie gardening might be something you've been meaning to do for some time. It might be something you've always wanted to try but never really knew where to start or how to go about it. It might seem impractical because you have pets that could damage the gardens, or because you are renting and might have to move on. There can be many impediments to taking the first step towards growing your own fruit and veggies at home.

The information in this section is designed to help you overcome all these impediments to getting started. Once you have that first plot dug, you will love getting out there on your own or as a family, learning new skills and growing your own fresh ingredients. Your homegrown veggies will taste sensational, save you money, give you a great sense of achievement and be an inspirational source of unusual produce to fuel your new healthy, active lifestyle.

Get to know your soil

The first thing you need to learn about before you engage in any type of gardening is your dirt! Literally. Once you've made the effort to get down and dirty in your garden you can begin to understand what your soil is all about. It is, after all, one of the most important factors (along with water and sunlight) in establishing and maintaining a healthy vegetable garden.

Soil is the first thing and the last thing you should think about whenever you start a new garden, improve an existing one or plant a shrub or a tree.

A good way to distinguish what type of soil you have is to grab a handful, moisten it lightly with water and knead it in your hands for a minute or so, then attempt to roll it into a ball. Generally speaking, if it holds the shape well and feels a bit like playdough, it is more of a heavy clay soil; if it refuses to be moulded, and crumbles or falls apart, it is a sandy soil.

Why is this important? While there is nothing intrinsically wrong with clay or sandy soil, neither is ideal for gardening. The type of soil you have will impact heavily on what you grow, how you water your gardens and what needs to be done to improve it for more successful vegetable gardening.

All types of soil benefit enormously from the addition of organic matter like compost, mushroom compost and products such as blood and bone and animal manure (see page 106). There are all sorts of pre-packaged products on the market (ask the staff at your local plant nursery for advice) or you can compile your own (see page 103 for instructions on making your own compost).

Understanding pH
It isn't as complicated as it may seem (really).

The term 'pH' stands for 'potential hydrogen'. In gardening terms, it tells us about the acidity or alkalinity of soil. The pH scale goes from 0 to 14, with 7 being neutral. 0 is an extremely acid pH, while a pH of 14 is extremely alkaline. If a soil is too acidic or too alkaline certain nutrients can become 'locked up' and are then unavailable to the plants, meaning that those plants will fail to thrive.

Most veggies enjoy a pH of around 6.5. However, there are exceptions, so it is always a good idea to do a little research on the pH requirements of any plant you are thinking of adding to your gardens.

The easiest way to check your soil's pH level is with a testing kit. You can buy them inexpensively from most nurseries and garden centres and they are very simple to use. Alternatively, and especially for larger scale pH testing, you can have it checked professionally by a company or university.

Composting

Adding compost is a great way to improve any soil type and boost the overall health of your garden. In fact, compost is like gold for your garden and helps the environment too!

Compost encourages earthworms, beneficial bacteria and micro-organisms that aerate the soil resulting in strong root growth and hardier plants. Compost has a very high nutritional value enabling plants to obtain vital foods for healthy growth and therefore helping them to be more resilient, and resistant to pests and diseases.

A soil rich in composted material has greatly improved water retention capabilities and plants grown in these conditions are noticeably less stressed between waterings. There will also be a general reduction in the quantity of water required.

You can buy compost from garden centres and nurseries, but it's very easy and cheap to make your own – it really only costs a little of your time. Starting a compost heap or bin allows you to recycle all your fruit and vegetable scraps, thus returning them to the earth in a natural healthy way.

Making your own compost

Composts vary a great deal depending on the materials used, the season, the local climate, moisture level and so on. I suggest starting with a basic formula before experimenting with your own personal tailored variety.

While you can set aside an area in the backyard for a compost heap, there are also many excellent bins and tumblers commercially available in a wide range of styles and sizes. Bokashi bins are great for those with limited time or space and they will provide you with an excellent source of fertiliser in return for your kitchen scraps. Worm farms are another efficient and fascinating option.

No matter where you live, there is a way you can turn your kitchen refuse into garden gold for your plants at next to no cost, other than a small amount of your time.

How it works. Composting is a naturally occurring process that relies on micro-organisms like bacteria, fungi, insects and worms to break down the organic material you put in the compost heap or bin. In the process, a lot of heat is generated. Temperatures can rise above 60°C in the centre of a compost heap and these high temperatures kill most (but not all) of the things you don't want in your compost (like weed seeds, insect larvae and nematodes).

What to include. A compost heap or bin should never be used as a dump. But it will happily process all fruit and vegetable scraps (cooked or raw), and non-flesh kitchen scraps such as bread, pastry, pasta, grains, legumes, and so on. Kitchen scraps should always be balanced out with carbonaceous materials like grass clippings, shredded paper, ripped up cardboard, hay, sawdust, dead leaves, legumes, sugar cane and straw, at a general rate of 10 carbonaceous material to 1 kitchen scraps.

Avoid adding weeds that have gone to seed as well as really tough weed types like nut grass. Some people add meat scraps, but you might prefer to avoid them as they can attract vermin and flies, resulting in foul odours or maggots in the compost.

Managing your composter. While your bin or heap is filling, try to make sure there are alternating layers of kitchen scraps and carbonaceous material. Always let a new batch of compost sit for three or four days once the bin is full. Turn it approximately once a day thereafter to allow it to aerate, as oxygen is a vital part of the process. (Use a garden fork to turn a compost heap, or rotate/tip your composting bin.)

Compost should always be kept moist but never soaked. (You will need to cover your compost heap with a tarp in times of heavy rainfall.) Compost that is too wet will give off a foul odour and compost that is too dry will decompose very slowly indeed. An old gardeners' trick is to grab a good handful of your compost (not right from the edge, but remember that it can be extremely hot in the middle) and squeeze it hard. It should feel slightly moist, and a very small amount of liquid should dribble out. If you need to add moisture try spraying the surface of the compost with water, or a weak solution of seaweed or fish emulsion for extra oomph.

Speeding up the process. Accelerators can be added to help your compost decompose more swiftly. There are commercial types available or you can use things like bran, yeast, yogurt or watered down molasses. Use only small amounts, proportionate to the size of your compost.

Dry leaf matter adds phosphorus and other trace elements, depending on the type, and can speed things up. Dolomite can be added for its trace elements. Wood ash and charcoal in small amounts can add nutrient value and improve drainage and aeration.

Experiment with different proportions of the various things you put into your compost until you have worked out the best mixture for your climate and conditions.

Mulching

I cannot stress enough the importance of a good mulch on your garden. It is worth its weight in gold! So what is it? Mulch is any kind of material, usually natural or organic, laid over the soil of your garden, around the plants, as a protective covering.

Mulch has so many benefits, one of the most important being to help your garden retain moisture, thereby reducing water usage. By protecting the soil surface, it aids soil stability and helps reduce fluctuations in the soil temperature. A good covering of mulch also encourages beneficial predatory insects and wildlife like lizards, helping to reduce pest insect populations that could otherwise wage war on your produce.

Always water your garden before applying mulch, and water the mulch down really well once it has been spread. Never put mulch thickly around or up against the trunk or stems of your plants – always leave some space for air circulation.

In addition to its many practical benefits, mulch can also be an attractive feature of your garden. Visit your local garden centre or nursery to look at options like coloured pebbles, natural stones, decorative stone chips, various types of gravel and dyed rocks.

A 'living mulch', in the form of a dense low-growing groundcover, can also be a very viable, low-maintenance and attractive option.

For dedicated vegetable growers, mulches such as sugar cane, tea tree, lucerne, straw and hay are excellent.

Fertilising

For best results, use a combination of slow-release and quick-release fertilisers on your garden.

Slow-release fertilisers include compost, manures, blood and bone, and slow-release fertiliser pellets. They are usually high in trace elements and give the plants a slow steady source of nourishment for stronger growth. Add them to the soil before planting, and at key points in the growing process, making sure they are evenly spread and well combined with the soil to avoid clumping and nutrient build-up.

Fast-release fertilisers most often come in liquid form (often mixed with water) and are generally sprayed or sprinkled onto the leaves of your plants with a spray-bottle or watering can. The many different brands usually include seaweed extract, fish emulsion or worm casting liquid.

I strongly recommend watering in newly planted seedlings and fruit trees with a weak solution of fish emulsion. Not only will it give them a good head start, it also helps to reduce the stress of transplanting, frost, salt spray, insect attacks and harsh climatic conditions. A weak solution is safe to use on all plants, including natives.

Positioning

Fruit and vegetables prefer positions where they are in full sun for the greatest possible number of daylight hours. Good drainage is important to most plants, so you should take the time to improve this by adding compost and other organic material to the soil before planting.

Companion planting involves growing plants together that either support one another, enjoy the same conditions or have are beneficial to each other. There are many books and courses devoted to this subject and it is well worth exploring, as having even a basic understanding of what to plant with what can really improve results in your garden. There are many plants that are great at repelling unwanted garden pests by exuding strong scents or chemicals. These can be planted near plants that are more susceptible to attack. At the other end of the scale there are those that attract beneficial garden predators to protect vegetables planted in their vicinity. Strong smelling herbs and plants like lavender and marigolds are great for repelling garden pests. Native flowering shrubs like callistemons and grevilleas will attract lots of beneficial birds and insects.

Creating ponds, artistically piling up rocks and logs to form hiding places, installing bird feeders and nesting boxes and applying thick layers of natural mulch will also attract helpful wildlife including lizards and frogs to your garden.

Never assume that vegetables are something you grow only in the confines of the backyard veggie patch. Far from it – there are so many beautiful looking edible plants that make a most interesting and aesthetic display.

Fruit and vegetables can be planted in all sorts

of places around the home provided the conditions are right. Consider using them to line driveways, brighten up flower beds, nestle among and beneath large established plants. Or plant them as a feature in window boxes and pots, especially in small gardens and on balconies. You can even plant veggies around your letterbox!

Let your imagination run wild. The possibilities are endless when you put your mind to it. Here are a few ideas to get you started:

- **Lettuces** planted en masse in mixed colours look fantastic as a bold edging display plant.
- **Capsicums** in a neat, tightly planted hedge look fabulous, with their dark green leaves and splashes of colourful fruit.
- **Cherry tomatoes** grown espalier-style on trellising with the lower leaves removed look striking, with the tomatoes dangling down from the green canopy like bunches of grapes (my neighbours and visitors have always found this a fascinatingly novel concept).
- **Silverbeet,** rainbow silverbeet and herbs like rocket and parsley always add a burst of lush green and colourful growth to any garden. They look gorgeous among roses and other flowers.
- **Eggplant** is another overlooked yet very attractive plant, with its glossy purple fruit and olive green leaves. It can form a dramatic centrepiece in a garden display or front garden bed. Try surrounding

it with white alyssum, chives and a blue-flowering groundcover like evolvus.

- **Onions** can be quite ornamental in the home garden and also work wonders to help protect other more fragile plants from insect attacks by masking their scents. Their flowers are most unusual and quite striking.

- **Chives** make for a really cute tufty edging plant and when they do eventually flower, the flowers are very pretty. Intermingle chives with other small grasses of different colours and textures and you have an attractive, highly scented display.

- **Strawberries** look gorgeous in terracotta pots (you can buy special strawberry pots), or dangling their lush fruit from hanging baskets.

- **Watermelon and pumpkin** can create great temporary groundcovers (with delicious results), for large areas prone to weeds.

- **Passionfruit,** a true favourite with many children and adults alike, is very easy to grow. It is a great plant for growing over ugly walls and fences but it also makes a delightful cover or shade provider when grown over a garden arch or gazebo, and the flowers are spectacular. Passionfruit vines can also be grown alongside other flowering or scented climbers for extra wow factor or to totally cover a long fence.

- **Citrus tree topiaries,** when grown along driveways in a long line of matching pots, have a classic and stylish look. Their flowers are deliciously scented and they look great in every season.

- **Tamarillo trees** are very aesthetically appealing.
- **Paw paws** add a real touch of that tropical oasis feeling.
- **Bananas** might look messy by themselves, but plant a tropical theme garden around them and visitors will think they've stumbled into a lost jungle paradise.
- **Pineapples** are wonderfully ornamental, hardy and sophisticated in any garden situation – as a feature, mass planted, or dazzling in a fantastic pot. They create a real talking point with visitors when they fruit in their second year.

There really are so many planting possibilities for fruit and vegetables, most of which are attractive in their own right. Don't hide them away in the confines of the backyard veggie patch – they should take pride of place in your gardens as the amazing and gorgeous plants they are.

Watering
Depending on the scale of your vegetable gardening, your watering plan can range from a watering can to a drip irrigation system. Try to water as early in the morning as possible, as this is a time of low water evaporation and it will help to reduce fungal problems such as mildew. Your plants will be able to face the upcoming day fresh and strong before dealing with the effects of the day's weather. Avoid watering the leaves of most vegetables, especially cucumber, pumpkin, zucchini, tomatoes and melons.

Water is always best applied at the base of the plant, or direct to the root zone. It is much more beneficial to give your plants (excluding seedlings) a long, slow, deep drink three to four times per week rather than a quick shallow one every day. Watering this way encourages stronger, deeper root growth and hardier plants.

Keeping the gardens well watered can be difficult, especially if you live in an area where there are strict water restrictions. But by being a bit creative, planning ahead and following some of the tips below and on pages 113–114, you can do it. Don't let a limited water supply put you off growing your own fruit and vegetables.

Water saving tips

- **Use grey water** from your washing machine. Have a grey water system and diverter hose installed – a visit to your local hardware store will give you a wide range of options, as well as advice on all the relevant regulations, equipment and methods. Use a garden-friendly detergent in your washing machine – it will act as a wetting agent, enabling the soil to absorb more moisture, thus preventing wasteful run-off.

- **Bucket out the bath water** after the kids have had a bath (this is also great exercise for the upper arms).

- **Use rain water** if you can. Install a tank, even if it's only a small one, purely for watering the garden.

- **Mulching** really improves the water-holding capabi-

---

lities of your gardens and helps to reduce plant stress. It also increases microbial activity that improves root growth and aeration of the soil, resulting in stronger plants with more efficient root systems that are better able to reach more sources of moisture. It reduces evaporation, and prevents the growth of weeds that will steal a lot of any water you do supply.

- **Improving the organic matter content** in your soil will really increase your gardens' moisture-holding capabilities.
- **Keep some buckets in your bathroom** and one at a time fill them up while you are in the shower (be careful not to allow any garden unfriendly products like commercial soaps and shampoos flow into the buckets with the water).
- **Water wisely.** If you can, restrictions permitting (it is always wise to check with your local council), invest in a good quality soaker or seeping hose. They are much more effective than large fan sprays or sprinklers at getting the water deep into the soil. They offer a slow method of watering that is more accurate and has less wastage.
- **Water early in the morning** if possible – this really is the best time to water your plants. There's less evaporation and a reduced risk of fungal diseases and problems.
- **Use water spikes.** These are a great little invention available from most hardware stores and garden centres. You just push them into the ground near the

root zone of the plant and attach an upside down, clean soft drink bottle full of water. It will slowly water the plant for you. These are also great if you are going away for the weekend.

- **Grow plants together.** Plants really do like companion-ship. They will always do better when grown as a little community, even in a grouping of pot plants with their own mini micro climate. They support one another and are stronger together.

- **Be ready for rain.** When you do get some of that precious rain, have containers in your backyard ready to catch whatever excess you can. This can even be a few buckets, or a kiddies' paddling pool, *but be sure never to leave young children unsupervised around any source of water.*

- **Strengthen your plants** by feeding them regularly with fish emulsion or seaweed extract. This will help to keep them less stressed between waterings and in drying weather conditions.

- **Don't over-fertilise,** particularly with the more synthetic and high-nitrogen types of fertilisers, as this can encourage really fast but soft, flimsy new growth that requires a lot of water to maintain it well.

Growing food in pots

The art of growing fruit trees and vegetables in pots and containers is a very old one, and has its origins in many different cultures and countries. Growing edible plants in pots around your home or business is both decorative and practical, especially for the busy working person or those with limited garden space and those renting.

There are a few general guidelines to follow and then you can let your imagination take over to create your own portable, edible paradise.

Sizing

When selecting pots always go for as large and as practical as you can afford. Generally, the larger the pot, the more water retention and nutrient availability there will be for your plant.

The look

Consider what style or theme you want and try to stick to it, as this will give your potted garden a much more finished and stylish look. Consider, for example, a grouping of dark blue glazed pots with plenty of lush green foliage; a selection of terracotta pots from smooth to ribbed, round, square and triangular – but all terracotta and earthy; a mix-and-match display of cheerful yellow and lime green glazed pots from really tiny to giant sized; or a selection of black and grey smooth glazed pots near a dark grey outdoor setting, complemented by brightly coloured plants both edible and ornamental, equally bright cushions and multicoloured solar powered lights.

View your outdoor space as another room of your home. Coordinate your outdoor furniture and ornaments with your garden and potted plants to achieve a really wondrous space where you will enjoy spending time.

Consider, too, whether you will need to move your pot plants around, as this can be a really important factor when deciding between, say, a plastic look-alike terracotta pot or the real thing (which is much heavier).

Getting set up

Once you have thought about the placement of your potted garden and how you might like it to look, there are some practical issues to consider before you invest in the pots, the potting mix and the plants. Different kinds of pots have different pros and cons – it's easy to be swayed by pots that look gorgeous but don't really meet your requirements.

Here are some basics to think about:

- **Terracotta pots** are very porous and can dry out quickly, leaving a few centimetres of hardened potting mix at the base. If you love the terracotta look, consider using a pot sealer (available from garden centres, hardware stores and plant nurseries) on the inside of the pots before planting. Use a rich potting mix with high moisture-holding qualities and good drainage capabilities. Remember that terracotta pots are relatively heavy, and large ones will be difficult to move once they're full of soil.
- **Plastic pots** are versatile and relatively light, but can hold moisture around the base. Consider

putting a thin layer (about 1 centimetre deep) of coarse washed sand at the very bottom of really large plastic pots to improve drainage.

- **Glazed pots** tend to be thin on the sides. Use a potting mix that contains a good amount of organic matter to help protect plant roots from summer heat.

- **Drainage holes** should be the first thing you look at when selecting your pot, regardless of what it is made of. There should be a good number of holes for the size of the pot and they should not be concentrated in one area.

- **Always use the best quality potting mix** you can find for potted plants. Trying to save a few dollars will only cost you more in the long run and your plants will never do as well as they could. The potting mix should be well aerated, light, rich and loamy and feel really healthy and vibrant when you run it through your fingers. Most good quality mixes already contain some fertiliser so you won't need to add any at the time of planting. Remember, a little fertiliser goes a long way in the confines of a pot, and it is better to underfeed the plants rather than risk burning by feeding them too much. Don't be tempted to use soil from the garden in pots; always use potting mix.

- **Mulch** around the top of your pot once you've planted. Be careful not to choke the stem or trunk of the plant.

Edible potted delights

The are so many options when it comes to edible gardening in pots. Here are some of my favourites:

- **Hanging strawberry baskets.** Really attractive and easy to harvest. Use a very rich potting mix, water regularly and plant a variety of strawberries. I really like the year-round fruiting types like Atlanta, as well as some of the more unusual varieties like Sweetie and Hokowasi.
- **Rainbow silverbeet in a big pot.** Always looks lush, and is easy to grow if you plant it in a big, deep pot and use premium potting mix. Versatile in so many recipes, silverbeet is a good source of iron and other nutrients.
- **Pots of chillies.** Some varieties are so attractive you won't want to eat them. And be warned: once you start growing chillies, they can become a real passion – there are so many types, colours and degrees of hotness that a chilli collection can become enormous!
- **Bowls of greens.** By using a really big pot or tub and mass-planting a variety of Asian greens, lettuces and small-growing salad greens including English spinach, you can achieve a fantastic effect, with different foliages blending together to make a real statement. The mixed greens are tasty, highly nutritious and incredibly versatile.
- **Dramatic pineapples.** A tall, modern, glazed pot adorned with a pineapple plant makes for an

aesthetic statement that oozes good taste and style. They look fantastic as the feature at a doorway or as a pigeon pair either side of an entranceway.

- **Capsicums on show.** With lush green foliage and the brilliance of red, purple, green or yellow fruit, capsicums look great in any outdoor setting and are probably one of the most widely eaten decorative plants.

- **Mushrooms in a trough.** Got a dark spot? Buy a mushroom kit (in season). Remove the kit intact and relocate it into your decorative pot of choice – long rectangular trough types work well. Keep the trough out of the sun and lightly spray it with water as required to keep the soil moist. You will have a lovely fresh supply of delicious mushrooms and a real talking point at your next barbecue.

- **Pots of parsley.** Parsley is easy to grow in a pot, so long as the pot is deep. Both the curly and flat-leaf (Italian) varieties have pretty foliage as well as being highly nutritious. Parsley is a welcome addition to many recipes, so it's a good idea to have a pot or two just outside the kitchen.

- **Tufts of chives.** Great for filling those small pots, tufts of chives make cute displays. Include some in a children's pot plant garden, on a windowsill, or to add interest to your outdoor table. Place them among other plants as a pest deterrent as well.

- **Flowering herbs** like lavender and rosemary are classics for a pot plant garden, and with good reason

– they are attractive, useful, hardy and very water wise.

- **Hanging herbs.** Fill hanging baskets with thyme, oregano, lemon thyme, mint, chocolate mint, Vietnamese mint (tastes a lot like coriander) and marjoram. Their delicious fragrances will waft around your outdoor spaces and, if they're near doorways or windows, right through your house.

- **Trellised or espaliered tomatoes.** Planting into a really large pot, why not cover a sunny wall of boring fence with an espaliered tomato? Or create a triangular teepee with three stakes and train your tomato around them – very popular with children.

- **Topiaries of fruit trees.** Pots are ideal for planting topiary trees – that is, trees you trim into interesting shapes. They look good singly, planted in a cluster of matching pots, or in a row of pots lining a driveway or path. Citrus are my favourite topiary trees as they have a beautiful fragrance, scented flowers, brightly coloured fruit and year-round lush green leaves. The varieties I like best are Lemon Meyer, Lemonade tree, Imperial mandarin, Variegated cumquat, Emperor mandarin and Tahitian lime, although many varieties are suitable, and new hybrid dwarf types are being released all the time. Have a chat with your local nursery person about what is best suited to your area and climate. Pruning plays a big part in managing your topiary trees, so arm yourself with the necessary tools. Giving the tree a good hard prune approximately once a year will produce vigorous and healthy growth, and the removal of unwanted 'arms' will help to maintain the desired shape and improve fruiting and access. Once you have established the preferred shape of your tree, only light maintenance such as thinning out should be required on a regular basis. Remember always to leave enough older wood for fruit bearing and structure.

Remember, whatever the plants in your pots, all will benefit from regular applications of a foliar fertiliser like fish emulsion or seaweed extract. Most need the occasional addition of a slow-release fertiliser as well.

Edible gardening projects

Once you get fully involved in the pram diet lifestyle, you might want to think about taking on a creative gardening project. Not only will it help keep you fit – it will also engage your ingenuity and imagination while providing fresh food for your kitchen.

In this section, there are detailed instructions for two edible gardening projects – a hanging herb garden, and fresh salad in a pot. Or you might like to let your imagination loose and come up with projects of your own.

Project 1: Hanging herb gardens

Herbs have so many uses and are generally very easy to grow. They are attractive, aromatic, a wonderful addition to many recipes, and a valuable asset in every garden.

In cooking, herbs add a tantalising array of flavours and scents, enhancing numerous meals and foods. When it comes to food, herbs can turn the ordinary into the extraordinary, as well as greatly reducing the need for added salt, sugar and saturated fats. In the garden, they release amazing aromas and range from thick, hardy groundcovers to beautiful fragrant flowers to useful trees and shrubs. They are excellent at repelling unwanted garden visitors and also at attracting beneficial garden friends.

They have an abundance of uses ranging from cooking, companion planting, decorating, medicinal properties and practical uses around the home to beauty treatments. A visit to your local bookstore or library, or a browse of the Internet, will provide you with a wealth of information about uses for herbs.

One easy way to get started on bringing herbs into your life is to grow a few of the basics. And one of the easiest ways of growing herbs is in hanging baskets. This is a perfect option for those who live in flats or units with balconies, have limited space, those who rent or even people whose family pets have a habit of digging in the garden. Most herbs (there are exceptions, so always refer to the label or advice from your local nursery person) enjoy good drainage, a lot of sunlight, not too rich a soil, and 'drying out' between fairly regular waterings.

To create your very own hanging herb garden, you will need:

- Some hanging baskets. Look for strong baskets that have adequate drainage holes. The wire-framed ones lined with coconut fibre are very effective; or look for deep plastic hanging pots. Avoid any that are very small or only have a few small drainage holes. Your hanging garden will look much more attractive if you choose hanging baskets or pots that are all the same, or stick to a theme.
- Hooks for hanging your baskets. A trip to your local hardware store or plant nursery will reveal a wide range of hooks and ways of attaching hanging baskets to walls, fences, verandahs, pergolas, trellises, window sills, balcony railings and eaves.
- A good quality potting mix – the foundation of successful gardening in containers. There are many types on the market, including some specifically intended for pots and planters and herbs.
- A watering can.
- Fish or seaweed emulsion.
- A selection of herbs suitable for growing in hanging baskets. It's best to buy punnets of healthy-looking seedlings. If you are unfamiliar with herbs, start with some easy-to-grow well-known varieties – your local nursery can advise you. These could include thyme,

oregano, common mint, chocolate mint, apple mint, peppermint, Vietnamese mint (used like coriander) and marjoram. Dwarf rosemary and dwarf lavender are also good options, but they will need larger, deep pots.

Setting up your hanging herb garden

1. Before establishing your hanging herb garden, find the ideal spot for it and plan the layout. There should be plenty of sunlight throughout the day, easy access (so that you can tend and water the herbs), and protection from wind and heavy rain. Ideally, your herb garden should be conveniently close to your kitchen. Remember that water will drain from the hanging pots or baskets, so check what is going to be underneath them. If you are concerned about draining water, consider positioning potted plants under the hanging baskets or using hanging pots with attached trays (these will need to be flushed occasionally and the trays checked for fungus and pests).

2. Soak your new herb seedlings in a very weak solution of fish emulsion for approximately 2–3 minutes.

3. Fill each of the hanging baskets with potting mix and arrange the drained seedlings on top of the soil to work out what you want to plant with what.

4. Plant the seedlings into the baskets, following directions on plant labels and any other relevant advice, but also being creative. Water them thoroughly.

Caring for your hanging herb garden

- Water regularly but be careful not to waterlog or over-water your herbs. Always check the potting mix with your finger to a depth of at least 3 centimetres to feel whether it is already moist. Some hanging baskets and pots can really hold moisture in that bottom layer, causing drainage problems, fungal diseases and root rot.

- Check for insect problems occasionally, although most herbs are reasonably trouble free when grown on a small scale.

- Fertilise the young plants with liquid fertiliser approximately once a fortnight until they are well established, then once a month with liquid fertiliser or approximately twice a year with slow-release fertiliser (always refer to the manufacturer's labelling). Note: it is *always* better to under-fertilise plants, particularly herbs, than to overdo it.

- Pick and use herbs as you need them for cooking, and enjoy their sensationally fresh flavour and aroma.

- Brighten up your house by adding a vase of scented herbs to a room. Or research the many non-culinary uses for various herbs — you'll be amazed at the creative and beneficial options your hanging herb garden offers you.

Project 2: Fresh salad in a pot

Why should you grow at least some fresh produce at home? And why is it a great idea to involve your children?

Growing your own produce brings you into real contact with real foods. It saves you money, provides you with a source of wonderfully fresh organic ingredients, and gives you a reason to be outside enjoying the fresh air. Gardening is great exercise and a good way to unwind and de-stress. Once you start growing your own food you will feel inspired to eat more fruits and vegetables and to use them more regularly in your cooking and day-to-day life.

Children gain a great sense of achievement and creative accomplishment, as well as learning practical skills and environmental awareness. Growing their own fruit and veggies is like a live science lesson, as well as being lots of fun. Children who get involved in organic gardening learn how to identify and photograph insects and wildlife, how the food chain works, and how plants interact with the rest of the natural world. They learn many lessons about taking responsibility and can take pride in knowing that they are contributing to a cleaner, healthier environment.

Anyone can succeed at growing delicious fresh ingredients — you just need some simple, easy-to-follow instructions, the right equipment and your own willingness to put in the effort.

When you first grow fresh produce it's a good idea to start small and not overload yourself. Start with one or two simple projects and build from there.

To grow your own salad-in-a-pot, you will need:

- One or more large, deep plastic pots (the bigger the better), with plenty of drainage holes in the bottom (this should be your first priority).
- A small amount of coarse sand to thinly line the base of each pot before adding the potting mix (it will improve drainage).
- A really good quality potting mix (it's important not to economise here because this will be the growing medium for your plants).
- A punnet each of soft-leaved, preferably non-hearting types of mixed lettuce like mignonette or coral; mixed salad greens like endive, Asian salad greens and rocket; English spinach; chives; and some flowers like pansies (in season) or marigolds. (For beginner gardeners or those with limited time it is better to start with punnets rather than seeds.)
- Some seaweed or fish emulsion liquid fertiliser.
- A watering can.

Setting up your salad-in-a-pot

1. Find a flat spot for your pot/s in a sunny position, preferably sheltered from strong winds. Ideally, when growing salad greens, you want the pot/s to be in the full sun for at least six hours a day for optimum plant growth and health. If you are growing your salad in a hot climate or in strong summer heat, place them under the protection of a light shade cloth through which they will still receive sun all day long.

2. Position your pot/s exactly where you want them. They can be heavy and difficult to move once established, so be sure it is somewhere convenient and practical. Next, consider what surface your pot will be sitting on. If it is coarse gravel or sand the pot/s will be well drained and aerated, but if they are going to be sitting on concrete, pavers or any other hard surface you may want to invest in some 'pot feet' for your pot to sit on. These can also be a good idea if you are putting the pot onto garden soil, as the gap between the pot and the ground will help prevent garden pests and fungal problems from reaching your potted plants via the soil.

3. First, line the base of the pots with a thin layer (about 1 centimetre) of coarse, washed sand, then fill your pot with quality potting mix. It should have a healthy colour and texture and feel crumbly and rich between your fingers. Water it in so that it settles into the pot/s.

4. Fill a bucket with a really weak solution of the fish emulsion, remove the seedlings from their punnets and gently immerse them in the mixture for 2–3 minutes.

5. Gently arrange your seedlings on the surface of the pot/s in a way that you might want to plant them. It is important to avoid being too methodical with an organic, mixed salad greens pot garden – the 'mixed up' effect helps to protect the plants from insect attack. Strongly fragrant chives, spring onions

and other scented plants and herbs mask the more susceptible salad plants with soft edible leaves, 'hiding' them and confusing potential insect pests. Always read the basic instructions on the punnet label guides regarding sizes and planting, remembering that you will be harvesting them quite often so may not need quite as much room as they specify. Then plant out your pot/s.

6. Pour the bucket of weak emulsion into a watering can and water the new seedlings in well.

Caring for your salad-in-a-pot

- Check your pot/s each day. Look for caterpillars or snails and remove any you find. Be careful to leave garden friends like ladybirds and praying mantis. If your salad garden is 'under attack' you may want to try an organic pest repellent spray.

- Water early each morning if possible, or in the late afternoon. If you live in a particularly hot area or it's a hot dry season you may want to provide a thin layer of mulch like sugar cane, hay, straw or lucerne to help keep the pot from drying out too quickly.

- Feed with a weak solution of the fish or seaweed emulsion each week (try to pick a set day to avoid doubling up or missing a week).

- Check if any plants are growing more quickly than others. If this occurs you might want to relocate the plants that are being overshadowed, or thin out the faster growing varieties.

- Harvest your greens as you want to use them, ensuring you are using them in as fresh a state as possible. Harvest the outside leaves of lettuces first and don't be afraid to remove some excess foliage from the more vigorous varieties if they are overtaking the pot.

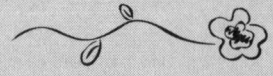

Eating The Pram
Diet Way

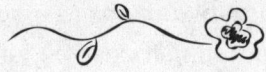

It is easy to overeat without realising that you have, simply by grazing on small amounts of foods constantly throughout the day. If you find it hard to walk past the fridge or pantry cupboard without opening the door then you probably aren't eating enough regular, filling meals. Having a menu plan in place allows you to see what and how much you are eating in a typical day. By eating healthy, wholesome meals and snacks at set points during the day you will keep your metabolism firing, improve your digestion and experience fewer cravings and binges. A structured eating plan will also ensure you are including plenty of fresh fruits and vegetables in your diet.

As well as improving your diet and thereby your health, a menu plan will allow you to streamline your weekly shopping and help you budget better. It's really important to shop with your menu plan in mind so that you have tasty, fresh ingredients handy, and some easy-to-make healthy snacks for those times when you are feeling peckish.

Because you draw up the menu plan yourself, it will eventually be tailor-made to suit your likes and dislikes, making it easy for you to stick to and ensuring that you don't skip meals and overeat later. Try to vary the plan from day to day so you don't get bored. And include a wide variety of healthy options to expand the range of healthy, energy-boosting foods you love to eat.

And remember: drink plenty of water every day, preferably not immediately before or after eating. Most health experts recommend at least eight glasses or about 2 litres of water daily to maximise body function and maintain healthy hydration.

DAILY MENUS

The following are some examples of my own daily menu plans. I constructed them myself, and know they work. You don't always have to eat the snacks or morning and afternoon teas, but if you include them in the plan you are completely covered for the day.

I have found that small light snacks keep my energy flowing and break up my mornings and afternoons. I've also noticed that by including a small amount of something 'not-so-healthy' in the day, usually for a snack or afternoon tea, I don't feel deprived and find it easier to stick to my plan – items like a few small squares of quality dark chocolate, a biscuit with afternoon coffee or a glass of red wine after dinner can actually help you to overcome any bad associations you might have had with food.

By eating small amounts of these foods once in a while, you will enjoy them more when you do consume them. It's all about balance:

- If you plan to have a small slice of cake at that birthday party, counter it by eating a really healthy breakfast, salad for your lunch, fruit for snacks that day and a healthy dinner of steamed vegetables and possibly a piece of grilled fish or chicken.
- When having takeaway dinner as a family, balance out the high-calorie foods with healthy ones. For example, for a family of four, instead of buying three large pizzas plus garlic bread and all eating large amounts, buy just one pizza and serve everyone a slice or two with plenty of fresh, tasty, dressed salad and homemade sweet potato wedges (you will save money as well as calories).
- When you're out and about and have to rely on takeaway food for a meal, swap those burgers and soft drinks for healthier options like a wholemeal falafel kebab with lots of salad and a sparkling mineral water, or fresh sushi and a freshly squeezed fruit juice. Eat really healthily for the rest of the day, make sure you get plenty of exercise, and you will still be leading a healthy lifestyle.

A week's worth of sample menu plans

DAY ONE

On rising

1 big glass of water with freshly squeezed lemon juice

Breakfast

1 small serve of Messy Mushrooms (page 152)
1 cup of coffee, tea or herbal tea with 1 teaspoon sugar
   (optional)

Morning tea

1 cup coffee, tea or herbal tea with 1 teaspoon sugar
   (optional)
2 low-fat choc-chip biscuits
1 big glass of water

Lunch

Fresh Italian-flavoured Salad (page 195)
1 glass of mineral water

Afternoon tea

5 squares of quality dark chocolate
1 big glass of water with freshly squeezed lemon juice

Dinner

1 small serve of Hearty Stockpot (page 184)

Dessert (optional)

small bowl of low-fat yogurt with ½ a fresh banana and
   5–8 blueberries

Additional snacks (optional)

water (as much as you like)
1 small orange or 2 small mandarins
a handful of almonds and sultanas

Alternatives

- Swap the Messy Mushrooms for Savoury Eggs on
  page 154.

- Swap the chocolate at afternoon tea for some
  cashews or some tomato salsa with celery and
  carrot sticks.

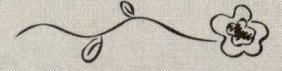

DAY TWO

On rising

1 big glass of water with freshly squeezed lemon juice

Breakfast

1 big glass of Watermelon Smoothie (page 156)

Morning tea

1 glass of mineral or tonic water

1 cup of coffee, tea or herbal tea (optional)

1 small Fibre Boost Choc Muffin (page 162)

Lunch

steamed sweet potato and organic carrot circles served
     with a tasty dressing

1 big glass of water

Afternoon tea

½ cup watermelon

½ cup rockmelon

a small handful of grapes

1 big glass of water

Dinner

oven-baked fish with crispy sweet potato wedges and
     Fresh Italian-flavoured Salad (page 195)

1 glass of red wine (optional)

Dessert (optional)

1 small serve of low-fat frozen yogurt with 4 squares quality dark chocolate shaved finely over the top

Additional snacks (optional)

water (as much as you like)
a handful of dried apricots and prunes
a handful of walnuts
1 apple

Alternatives

* Instead of fruit for afternoon tea, try crispbread with hummus or a cup of coffee and a chocolate biscuit.

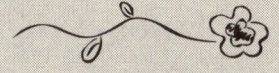

DAY THREE

On rising
I big glass of water with freshly squeezed lemon juice

Breakfast
I cup of coffee, tea or herbal tea with I teaspoon sugar
(optional)
I slice whole grain unbuttered toast with I mashed ripe
banana and a sprinkle of cinnamon

Morning tea
I apple and I nectarine, cut into cubes
I glass of water with freshly squeezed lemon juice

Lunch
Gorgeously Green Salad with fat-free French dressing
(page 158)
I big glass of mineral water

Afternoon tea
2 fat-free crackers with hummus, tabouleh and fresh
sprouts and (optional) tuna or ham

Dinner
a small serve of Tasty Tuna Rice (page 201)
I glass of red wine (optional)

Additional snacks (optional)

water (as much as you like)

1 glass of Watermelon Smoothie (page 156), with added phylum husks, flaxseed oil and LSA

a handful of raw unsalted mixed nuts

Alternatives

*   Try a healthy burger for dinner instead (see page 186).

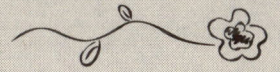

DAY FOUR

On rising
1 big glass of water with freshly squeezed lemon juice

Breakfast
1 bowl bircher-style or low-fat whole grain muesli (approximately ½ cup), with added phylum husks and ½ a fresh banana, chopped
1 glass of freshly squeezed orange juice, or water with freshly squeezed lemon juice

Morning tea
1 cup of coffee, tea or herbal tea with 1 teaspoon sugar (optional)
5 squares quality dark chocolate or 1 chocolate biscuit

Lunch
a small serve of Messy Mushrooms (page 152)
1 big glass of mineral water

Afternoon tea
1 cup of coffee, tea or herbal tea with 1 teaspoon sugar (optional)
a small serve of salsa with celery sticks, carrot sticks, capsicum slivers and rice crackers

Dinner

Perfectly Pizza with fresh Italian-style salad (see pages
    193 and 195)
1 glass of tomato juice
1 big glass of water

Additional snacks (optional)

water (as much as you like)
¼ cup rockmelon or honeydew melon
a handful of walnuts and 4–5 strawberries
1 cup of coffee, tea or herbal tea

Alternatives

• For a lighter dinner try the Roast Pumpkin and Feta
  Salad on page 175.

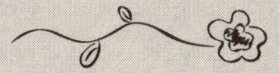

DAY FIVE

On rising
1 big glass of water with freshly squeezed lemon juice

Breakfast
freshly made fruit salad with low-fat custard
1 glass of water with freshly squeezed lemon juice

Morning tea
1 cup of coffee, tea or herbal tea with 1 teaspoon sugar
    (optional)
2 low-fat biscuits
1 big glass of water

Lunch
1 mountain bread wrap with fresh rocket, baby spinach
    leaves, shredded soft lettuce leaves, grated carrot,
    finely grated raw beetroot, tabouleh, hummus, low-fat
    feta cheese and (optional) tuna, skinless chicken or
    fat-free ham
1 big glass of mineral water

Afternoon tea
1 cup of coffee, tea or herbal tea with 1 teaspoon sugar
    (optional)
4 squares quality dark chocolate
a handful of sultanas, prunes, dried apricots and dates
    with a small handful of walnuts, pecans and almonds
1 big glass of water

Dinner

light fish portion with Avocado Whip (page 168) and freshly steamed veggies (including broccoli, carrots, green beans and Brussels sprouts)

Dessert (optional)

a small bowl of frozen yogurt or a frozen Watermelon Smoothie (page 156)

Additional snacks (optional)

water (as much as you like)

1 cup of low-fat soup

1 banana

Alternatives

* Have a small serve of Moist Pumpkin Cake (see page 166) for afternoon tea.

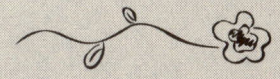

DAY SIX

On rising

I big glass of water with freshly squeezed lemon juice

Breakfast

I cup of coffee, tea or herbal tea with I teaspoon sugar (optional)

I small bowl low-fat yogurt with added LSA, phylum husks, flaxseed oil, a few blueberries and some chopped banana and nectarine

Morning tea

I cup of coffee or tea with I teaspoon sugar (optional)

I slice whole grain toast, unbuttered, with avocado, fresh tomato and freshly cracked black pepper

I big glass of water

Lunch

a small portion of Warm Sweet Potato Salad (page 177) with some steamed broccoli, cabbage and snow peas

I glass of mineral water

Afternoon tea

½ cup watermelon slices

I big glass of water

Dinner

I slice of Quick Asparagus Quiche (page 179) with lots of Fresh Italian-flavoured Green Salad (page 195)

Additional snacks (optional)

water (as much as you like)
4 squares quality dark chocolate
a small handful of almonds
1 glass of red wine

Alternatives

- Today you could try the Perfectly Pizza (on page 193) for dinner instead.

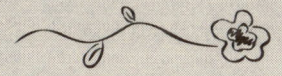

DAY SEVEN

On rising
1 big glass of water with freshly squeezed lemon juice

Breakfast
1 cup of coffee, tea or herbal tea with 1 teaspoon sugar
    (optional)
1 small serve scrambled eggs with added baby spinach,
    rocket, tomato, sliced snowpeas and grated zucchini,
    served with fresh sprouts and freshly ground black
    pepper

Morning tea
1 glass of water with freshly squeezed lemon juice
¼ cup rockmelon, ¼ cup watermelon and
    approximately 10 grapes

Lunch
fresh green salad with low-fat dressing and low-fat feta
    cheese
1 glass of mineral water

Afternoon tea
1 cup of organic white tea with 1 teaspoon honey
    (optional)
2 small biscuits

Dinner

1 bowl of low fat soup – sweet potato and lentil, homemade vegetable or pumpkin

1 wholemeal bread roll, warmed in the oven and spread with spicy low-fat dip or hummus (optional)

Additional snacks (optional)

water (as much as you like)

1 banana

1 small bowl low-fat yogurt

1 glass of vodka (a small nip) with tomato juice

Alternatives

- Serve a bowl of soup with a portion of Turkish Tempters (page 160), or instead try a dinner of Sprout Stirfry (page 206).

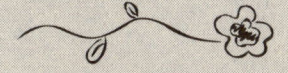

BREAKFAST RECIPES

EXOTIC HOLIDAY YOGURT
Serves 2

Ingredients
½ cup low-fat yogurt
1 tablespoon flaxseed oil
1 tablespoon finely ground almonds, sunflower seeds and hazelnuts (also available as LSA or 'Women's Nutrient Formula' from most supermarkets and health food stores)
1 banana, chopped
1 fresh, ripe plum or nectarine, chopped
½ cup rockmelon, chopped
3–4 ripe strawberries, thinly sliced
1 tablespoon shredded coconut

Method
1 Mix yogurt, flaxseed oil and ground nuts well.
2 Gently toss the chopped fruit through the yogurt mixture, ensuring it is well coated.
3 Serve in a chilled bowl topped with shredded coconut.

Notes
- This simple recipe is quick to make, versatile, healthy and appealing for you and your family.
- This is a really flexible recipe. Use a selection of whatever fruit is in season, or your own personal favourites.

- Excellent for entertaining. Serve in decorative, chilled bowls topped with fresh passionfruit and a very small amount of finely grated white chocolate.
- A perfect light breakfast for those who dislike feeling full and heavy in the mornings, those who are prone to skipping breakfast entirely and people who find it hard to include plenty of fresh fruit in their day.

Toddler tip

- Serve your toddler cubed fruit with a bowl of yogurt combined with a small amount of flaxseed oil or powdered baby cereal. This will make it a much thicker consistency and easier for them to eat. Most supermarkets now stock organic baby cereals which are around the same price as their non-organic counterparts.

- Experiment with differently flavoured low fat yogurts, or even try natural yogurt.

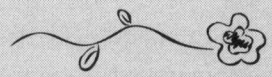

TRENDY TOMATO TOAST
Serves 4

Ingredients
4 slices whole grain bread
2 tablespoons hummus
½ cup fresh tabouleh
1 ripe avocado, cut into long thin pieces
1 fresh ripe tomato, thinly sliced
1 red onion, very thinly sliced
freshly ground black pepper
sea salt (optional)
fresh red chilli, very finely chopped (optional)

Method
1 Toast the bread and put it on a plate.
2 While the toast is still warm, spread it with the hummus, then top it with the rest of the ingredients, in layers.

Notes
- This recipe is really filling as well as being very tasty.
- It tastes best when made with fresh, bright red, beautifully ripe tomatoes (preferably organic).
- You can also add a thin slice of fat-free ham to each slice of toast as a first layer before the salad ingredients.

Toddler tip

- For toddlers or younger children, try spreading whole grain toast with a combination of hummus and cream cheese, or avocado and cream cheese and cut each slice into small squares or triangles. Depending on whether they like the texture or not, lightly sprinkle with tabouleh. Serve with some cubes of avocado, cherry tomatoes and fresh crunchy snowpeas.

- Try adding fresh pineapple slices and cooked skinless chicken for a different flavour.

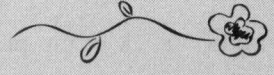

MESSY MUSHROOMS
Serves 4

Ingredients
2 teaspoons extra virgin olive oil
2 slices vegetarian soy rashers or low-fat bacon
500 grams mushrooms, sliced
½ cup broccoli, very finely chopped
1 tablespoon soy sauce
2 tablespoons light sour cream (or more to taste)
1 cup baby spinach leaves, shredded
freshly ground black pepper
chilli (optional)

Method
1 Heat the oil in a non-stick frying pan over medium heat.
2 Add the soy rashers or bacon and fry until lightly crisp, then add the mushrooms, broccoli and soy sauce. Stir gently until the mushrooms are soft and cooked through.
3 Stir in the sour cream and baby spinach leaves and cook for about 1 minute.
4 Sprinkle with freshly ground black pepper and chilli. Serve alone or on top of a slice of unbuttered whole grain toast.

Notes
• A perfect dish for lunch.
• Place small amounts on thin slices of lightly toasted

French stick (wholemeal if available) and serve as a hot entree.

- Add thin slivers of zucchini and capsicum as extra vegetables.
- Turn Messy Mushrooms into a main meal by increasing the ingredient quantities and adding a little extra sour cream to make more sauce. Serve on a bed of cooked brown rice with a small crusty wholemeal bread roll.

Toddler tips
- The tasty flavour is very appealing to children, even those who may 'dislike mushrooms'.

- Serve toddlers a cooled portion with some chunks of fresh wholemeal bread.

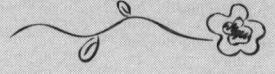

SAVOURY EGGS
Serves 4

Ingredients
1 teaspoon extra virgin olive oil
1 onion, finely chopped
2 spring onions, finely sliced
1 cup chopped ripe tomato
1 medium zucchini, finely grated
1 red capsicum, finely chopped
½ teaspoon paprika
½ teaspoon chopped fresh red chilli (optional)
freshly ground black pepper
sea salt
4 free range eggs
½ cup baby spinach leaves, chopped
2 teaspoons finely chopped fresh chives
3 teaspoons finely chopped fresh parsley
1 teaspoon dried thyme

Method
1 Heat the oil in a non-stick frying pan over medium heat, then add the onion and cook for 2 minutes or until it becomes translucent.
2 Add the spring onions, tomato, zucchini and capsicum and stir over medium heat for a further 2 minutes.
3 Sprinkle with some of the paprika and chilli, and season with freshly ground black pepper and a small sprinkle of sea salt. Reduce the heat to low.

4 Crack the eggs carefully into the mixture, then toss the baby spinach leaves, chives, parsley and thyme into the frying pan as well. Mix gently together.

5 Stir the mixture continuously but gently over low heat until the egg is well cooked but not rubbery.

6 Serve immediately, topped with a sprinkle of freshly ground black pepper, chives and paprika.

Notes

- This can be served on whole grain unbuttered toast.
- Low-fat ham or vegetarian soy rashers can be added with the onion for a different flavour.
- This recipe is very tasty with mushrooms added.
- The dish can be made with egg whites only, by whisking them with a little low-fat milk in a bowl before adding them to the pan.
- For a warming, comfort-style cooked breakfast serve baked beans and grilled tomato alongside.

Toddler tips

- Chop the vegetables very finely and add some grated cheese at the same time as you add the eggs.

- Serve with triangles of grilled cheese on toast.

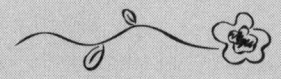

SNACKS AND FILLERS

WATERMELON SMOOTHIES
Serves 2

Ingredients
1 cup chopped watermelon (seedless or seeds
   removed)
1 banana, chopped
¼ cup chopped rockmelon
half a punnet of strawberries
¼ cup blueberries
¼ cup low-fat yogurt
1 tablespoon flaxseed oil
1 tablespoon phylum husks

Method
1 Place all ingredients in a blender and blend together
   thoroughly.
2 Serve in a tall glass with crushed ice (optional).

Notes
- A balanced healthy breakfast, especially for those who don't like a heavy start to the day or have a tendency to skip breakfast altogether.
- This refreshing and revitalising breakfast is great on busy days before going on a big walk or exercising.
- Easy to make for a whole family or to serve as a refreshment at a luncheon or dinner party.

- An achievable way of getting fresh fruit into your children's and your daily diet.
- A popular, healthy after-school pick-me-up that is very cost-effective when melons are in season.
- Try substituting other berries and fruits but keep the yogurt and additives base.
- Strain and serve in a decorative glass with shaved ice as a non-alcoholic cocktail.

Toddler tips

- Children love watermelon smoothies but they are quite thick. I suggest watering them down with some milk or soy milk for toddlers.
- Try mixing it with yogurt or organic powdered baby cereal for a thick and delicious breakfast for little ones, or even as an early food. This was my daughter's favourite breakfast when she was a baby – the watermelon gives it a very attractive colour which especially appeals to little ones.
- Freeze watermelon smoothie to make yummy, healthy icy poles (that adults love too).
- This can also be used to make a moist cake by adding 1 cup of smoothie to a mix of ¼ cup butter, ¼ cup sugar, 2 eggs and 2 cups of self-raising flour. Follow a basic cake method using a food processor.

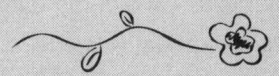

GORGEOUSLY GREEN SALAD
Serves 4

Ingredients
4 cups fresh salad greens, loosely packed
3–4 ripe organic tomatoes, diced or thinly sliced
¼ cup fresh sprouts (any kind)
1 ripe avocado, peeled, seed removed, and cubed
¼ cup sunflower seeds
¼ cup pepitas
2 spring onions, finely chopped
1 red onion, thinly sliced in rings
¼ cup finely grated fresh beetroot
¼ cup walnut pieces (optional)
¼ cup tasty salad dressing (fat-free Italian, French or honey-mustard, bought or homemade)

Method
1 Combine all the ingredients except the dressing in a large bowl.
2 Drizzle the dressing over the salad and toss to combine. Serve immediately.

Notes
- Any of the following can be added to this style of salad: almonds, sesame seeds, cashew nuts, cucumber, pineapple, grapes, sultanas, raw mushrooms, broccoli, snowpeas, capsicum, dates, pear, celery, all kinds of onion, low-fat feta cheese, small amounts of low-fat yellow cheese, fresh herbs.

- Always use fresh soft-leaved salad greens (rather than iceberg lettuce).
- Experiment with edible fresh greens like baby spinach leaves, fresh rocket, fresh coriander, mustard leaves and baby Asian greens.
- This is great dish for serving up fresh greens and produce from your garden.
- Increase the quantities to take as a prepared dish to a barbecue or dinner party.
- Serve as an accompaniment to main meals or as a tasty, healthy lunch.
- This salad is great with cold, cooked chicken or smoked salmon slices as a refreshing main meal in hot weather.

Toddler tip
- Prepare a separate toddler-friendly version while making the adult salad. Include cubes of fresh tomato, avocado, cucumber and cheese, fresh crunchy snowpeas, sweetcorn kernels, pineapple pieces and chopped hard-boiled eggs.

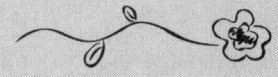

TURKISH TEMPTERS
Serves 4

Ingredients
2 long loaves low-fat Turkish bread
1 cup organic tomato paste
4 garlic cloves, crushed
1 cup baby spinach leaves
200 grams low-fat feta cheese, crumbled
1 tablespoon dried mixed herbs
freshly ground black pepper

Method
1 Cut the bread into pieces 10–15 centimetres long, and split each piece. Place the pieces split-side-up on a clean board or kitchen bench.
2 Spread each piece of bread with tomato paste, followed by a generous amount of garlic, then the baby spinach leaves. Top with a thin layer of crumbled feta cheese and sprinkle with herbs and black pepper.
3 Brown under a hot grill until the feta is melty and slightly coloured.
4 Serve immediately.

Notes
• Add a dash of chilli, slice of ham or a thin pineapple slice for a different flavour.
• Serve with lightly dressed fresh soft lettuce leaves and mixed sprouts for a quick, tasty lunch or light dinner.

- These are great with soup.
- Perfect fingerfood for entertaining.
- Experiment with different breads, like wholemeal rolls.
- Swap feta for low-fat cheddar cheese if preferred.

Toddler tip
- Try using yellow cheese if the feta flavour is too strong, and omit the pepper.

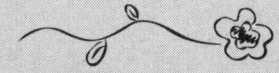

FIBRE BOOST CHOC MUFFINS
Makes 12

Ingredients
¼ cup butter, softened
2 teaspoons olive oil (optional, for extra moisture)
¼ cup raw sugar
2 free range eggs
1 cup low-fat yogurt
1 tablespoon honey
1 tablespoon cocoa, dissolved in hot water and
    allowed to cool
¼ cup dates, finely chopped
¼ cup walnuts, roughly chopped
¼ cup prunes, finely chopped
3 tablespoons LSA
2 tablespoons wheat germ
50 grams quality dark chocolate, melted
2 cups wholemeal self-raising flour, sifted
extra quality dark chocolate, shaved, for decorating

Method
1 Preheat the oven to 180°C (160°C fan-forced) and
   prepare 2 six-hole muffin trays by placing muffin
   liners in each hole.
2 In a large bowl combine the butter, olive oil and
   sugar until smooth and creamy.
3 Add the eggs, mix together, then add the yogurt
   and honey and mix well.

4 Add the cocoa, dates, walnuts, LSA, wheat germ, prunes and the melted chocolate and mix together.

5 Add the sifted flour and very gently mix it through until just combined. Pour into the muffin cases immediately.

6 Top each muffin with some grated dark chocolate.

7 Bake for 20 minutes or until the muffins spring back when gently touched and a toothpick comes out clean when inserted into the centre.

8 Remove the muffins to a wire rack, cover with a soft cloth and allow to cool.

Notes

- Using mini muffin trays and reducing the baking time will give you more serves but smaller portions.
- Muffins can be individually frozen and reheated in a microwave for a delicious instant snack or afternoon tea.
- Leave out the cocoa and melted chocolate and replace with finely-shredded coconut for a different flavour, and decorate with chopped dates.
- These can also be made with sultanas or cashews in the mix.

BEAN SALAD
Serves 4

Ingredients
450 gram can of three- or four-bean mix, rinsed and
    drained
1 white onion, finely diced
1 cup canned corn kernels, drained
1 red capsicum, finely diced
1 celery stick, finely diced
2 tablespoons of fat-free thousand island dressing,
    bought or homemade

Method
Combine all the ingredients in a medium-sized
    bowl, making sure the dressing is tossed through
    well.

Notes
- Serve as a side dish.
- Great as a topping over freshly steamed or mashed
  sweet potato.
- Perfect for entertaining, or to take to barbecues and
  dinner parties.
- Wonderful served with cold meats.
- Add a cup of chickpeas or red kidney beans, and
  try some extra dressing.
- This complements the Warm Sweet Potato Salad
  (page 177).

Toddler tip

- Set aside a toddler portion before you add the onion, and serve it with a selection of mashed or boiled baby potatoes, grilled fish or skinless chicken, strips of low-fat ham, chopped hard-boiled eggs, some chopped tomatoes and avocado cubes.

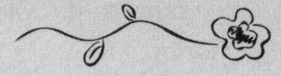

MOIST PUMPKIN CAKE
Serves 8–10

Ingredients
125 grams butter
½ cup raw sugar (or ¼ cup honey)
2 free range eggs
¾ cup low-fat or natural yogurt
1 cup mashed, cooked pumpkin, cooled
1 cup dates, finely chopped
¼ cup walnuts, chopped (optional)
2 tablespoons LSA (or finely ground almonds, linseed and sunflower kernels)
¼ teaspoon cinnamon
1 teaspoon lemon juice
2 cups wholemeal self-raising flour

Method
1 Preheat the oven to 180°C (160°C fan-forced).
2 Grease a 24 centimetre cake tin (which is at least 5 cm deep) and line the base with baking paper.
3 Combine the butter and sugar until soft and creamy.
4 Add the eggs one at a time, stirring until the mixture is smooth.
5 Mix in the yogurt followed by the pumpkin, dates, walnuts, LSA, cinnamon and lemon juice and combine well.
6 Sift in the flour, mix in well, then pour the mixture into the prepared cake tin.

7 Bake for 45 minutes or until the cake springs back when gently touched, is golden in colour and a skewer comes out clean when inserted into the centre.

Notes

- This cake is very soft and light and is delicious straight from the oven.
- A great way of using pumpkin if you have excess growing in your garden.
- Makes a delicious healthy birthday cake, drizzled with some melted white chocolate and walnut sprinkles.
- Enjoy a small portion as afternoon tea.
- Leave the walnuts out if you prefer your cakes nut-free, or swap the walnuts for pecans for a different flavour.
- Excellent for entertaining, especially when topped with lemon-flavoured icing.

Toddler tips

- Cut into small portions and frozen, this cake makes excellent quick snacks for your little one.
- Serve toddlers a small slice for afternoon tea with some chopped banana and pear.
- Leave out the walnuts and use the mixture to make mini muffins – great for children.

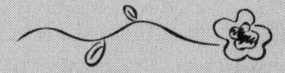

AVOCADO WHIP

Makes approximately 1½ cups

Ingredients

2–3 ripe avocados
¼ cup light sour cream
1 tablespoon sweet chilli sauce (or to taste)
freshly ground black pepper
fresh parsley to garnish

Method

1 Mash the avocados well with a fork or hand blender.
2 Stir in the sour cream and sweet chilli sauce.
3 Season with freshly ground black pepper and serve in a small bowl garnished with a sprig of fresh parsley.

Notes

- Great as a dip with rice crackers and freshly cut sticks of carrot, celery and red capsicum.
- Serve with some oven-baked sweet potato and carrot wedges.
- Use as a topping over lightly crumbed grilled fish or chicken.
- A delicious addition to mountain bread wraps with lots of fresh salad greens, crisp onion, grated carrot and sprouts.
- Spread on whole grain sandwiches as a healthy alternative to butter or mayonnaise.

- Replace the sour cream with natural yogurt if preferred.
- Serve in minature bowls, one per person, for an interesting dinner party entrée.
- Use as a topping for nachos.
- Great when freshly made for picnics.
- You can 'chunk it up' with pieces of chopped ripe tomato and celery.

Toddler tip
- Children love this dip. Serve them a bowl of it with plenty of celery and carrot sticks.

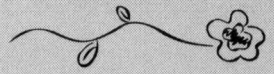

BANANA MUFFINS
Makes 12

Ingredients
¼ cup butter

¼ cup brown sugar

1 teaspoon vanilla essence

2 free range eggs

½ cup low-fat natural or vanilla yogurt

1 cup of mashed really ripe banana

1 grated pear

¼ cup raspberries

2 tablespoons LSA or a blend of ground almonds, sunflower kernels and linseed.

¼ cup wheat germ

¼ teaspoon baking powder

1 teaspoon cinnamon

¼ cup desiccated coconut

1 teaspoon raw sugar

1½ cups wholemeal self-raising flour, sifted

Method
1 Preheat the oven to 180°C (160°C fan-forced) and prepare 2 six-hole muffin trays by placing muffin liners in each hole.
2 In a bowl combine the butter and brown sugar until creamy.
3 Add the vanilla essence and the eggs, one at a time, stirring until the mixture is smooth.

4 Add the yogurt and mix in well, then add the banana, pear, raspberries, LSA, wheat germ, baking powder and cinnamon and mix them through.

5 In a separate small bowl combine the coconut and raw sugar, and set aside.

6 Add the sifted flour and very gently mix it through until just combined. Pour into the muffin cases.

7 Top each muffin with some of the sugar and coconut mix.

8 Bake for 15 minutes or until the muffins spring back when gently touched and a toothpick comes out clean when inserted into the centre.

9 Remove the muffins to a wire rack, cover with a soft cloth and allow to cool.

Notes

- For extra moisture increase the yogurt content slightly.
- Make the portions smaller by using mini muffin trays and reducing the baking time.
- You can add some white chocolate chips – but remember, they add extra calories.
- Substitute a sweet apple for the pear and blueberries or cranberries for the raspberries.
- Add ¼ cup chopped walnuts and dates for a different taste.
- For a special dessert, serve warm with low-fat custard, fresh chopped banana and shredded coconut.

Toddler tips

- These are best made as mini muffins for young children.

- To add colour and interest, top them with a sprinkling of hundreds and thousands instead of the sugar/coconut mix.

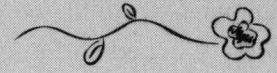

TUNA SALAD
Serves 4

Ingredients
¼ cup fat-free mayonnaise
1 teaspoon whole grain mustard
juice of ½ a lemon
1 teaspoon chopped fresh dill
400 gram can tuna in spring water, drained
½ cup canned corn kernels, drained
1 white onion, thinly sliced into rings
1 celery stalk, thinly sliced
2 ripe tomatoes, thinly sliced
½ small cucumber, finely sliced
¼ cup sunflower seeds
2 cups shredded rocket, loosely packed
1 ripe avocado, thinly sliced
parsley sprigs for garnishing
freshly ground black pepper

Method
1 Make the dressing by combining the mayonnaise, mustard, lemon juice and dill, and set aside.
2 In a medium sized bowl combine all the other ingredients except the avocado, parsley and black pepper.
3 Pour the dressing over the salad and stir through to lightly coat all the ingredients.
4 Serve on individual plates and top with thin slices of ripe avocado, sprigs of parsley and freshly ground black pepper.

Notes

- You can substitute salmon for the tuna.
- This is also delicious with a handful of mixed nuts added.
- Try serving alongside steamed vegetables and mashed pumpkin for a main meal or in a toasted, wholemeal, crusty bun topped with sesame seeds.
- For special occasions and entertaining, add some different seafood like cooked, peeled prawns and cooked crab meat, some sun dried tomatoes (not in oil), and increase the dressing.
- This is great in wholegrain sandwiches with lots of fresh salad greens.

Toddler tip

- Serve with mashed potato, mashed pumpkin, chopped hard-boiled egg and whole grain toast soldiers. Or try it as a filling with fresh soft lettuce in a wholemeal bun cut into toddler-friendly quarters.

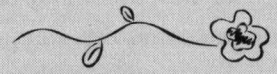

ROAST PUMPKIN AND FETA SALAD

Serves 4

Ingredients

½ a medium sized pumpkin

extra virgin olive oil for spraying

freshly ground black pepper

1 cup baby spinach leaves, loosely packed

½ cup rocket leaves, loosely packed

¼ cup sunflower seeds

¼ cup pepitas

200 grams low-fat feta cheese

1 red onion, finely sliced

1 small red capsicum, thinly sliced

1 celery stalk, thinly sliced

2 tablespoons low-fat honey-mustard dressing (bought or home-made)

Method

1 Preheat the oven to 180°C (160°C fan-forced).

2 Peel the pumpkin and chop it into bite-sized chunks.

3 Line a baking tray with greaseproof paper and a light spray of olive oil or use a non-stick tray. Place the pumpkin pieces on the tray, avoiding any overlapping.

4 Lightly spray the pumpkin with extra virgin olive oil and sprinkle with freshly ground black pepper.

5 Bake in the oven for 15 minutes or until golden and starting to crisp at the outside edges.

6 Meanwhile, tear the baby spinach and fresh rocket leaves into a large bowl and toss with the seeds.

7 Cut the feta into small cubes and lay them out on a baking-paper-lined tray.

8 Top the baby spinach and rocket mix with the onion, capsicum and celery slices and drizzle with the dressing.

9 Remove the cooked pumpkin from the oven and add to the salad while still warm.

10 Place the feta in a warm oven for 1 minute or until it is softened and warm (but not too runny or burnt).

11 Add the feta to the salad and gently toss it through until all the ingredients are well combined.

12 Serve immediately.

Notes
- Serve with a piece of grilled fish, lean meat, or skinless chicken for a healthy and very tasty main meal.
- Swap the dressing for a low-fat mayonnaise mixed with a little whole grain mustard and lemon juice.
- The quantities can be adjusted to make a single serving.
- Great to serve at a barbecue, dinner party and when entertaining.

Toddler tip
- Try serving your little one cooled pumpkin cubes with cubes of yellow cheese, strips of red capsicum, sticks of celery and fish nuggets (made from sustainably caught fish).

WARM SWEET POTATO SALAD
Serves 4

Ingredients
4 cups sweet potato, cut into bite-sized pieces
3 slices vegetarian soy rashers or low-fat bacon
¼ cup low-fat mayonnaise
1 onion, thinly sliced into rings (optional)
¼ cup pepitas
2 cups baby spinach leaves, loosely packed
freshly ground black pepper

Method
1 Place the sweet potato in a saucepan of boiling water, reduce the heat and simmer until just cooked so that a fork easily penetrates but the pieces don't fall apart. Drain and set aside.
2 Cut the soy rashers or bacon into very thin strips and spread them on an alfoil-lined baking tray. Grill or bake the bacon until it is crispy, then drain on paper towel and set aside.
3 In a large bowl, gently combine the warm sweet potato pieces with the mayonnaise, ensuring they are well coated. Then add the onion, pepitas and crispy bacon.
4 Divide the baby spinach leaves between four plates, and top with the sweet potato salad and freshly ground black pepper.

Notes

- For an even healthier version, you can leave out the bacon.
- A little mustard and a dash of freshly squeezed lemon juice will add more of a tang to the mayonnaise.
- Great for barbecues, entertaining and as a side dish.
- For something different, add 1 cup of cooked pumpkin or carrot chunks and a little extra dressing.
- This recipe can also be made with regular potato, or half and half with sweet potato.

Toddler tip
- Try using yellow cheese if the feta flavour is too strong, and omit the pepper.

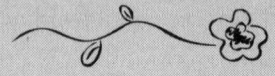

MAIN MEALS

QUICK ASPARAGUS AND
COTTAGE CHEESE QUICHE
Serves 4–6

Ingredients

1 sheet low-fat pastry (preferably wholemeal or whole grain), semi defrosted

1 bunch fresh asparagus, lightly blanched and chopped into small pieces, or 400 gram can asparagus pieces, drained

2 free range eggs

¼ cup low-fat cheese, finely grated

125 grams low-fat cottage cheese

¼ cup thinly sliced green or yellow capsicum

3 spring onions, sliced

1 teaspoon fresh red chilli, finely chopped (to taste)

1 teaspoon finely chopped fresh chives

1 teaspoon finely chopped fresh parsley

1 teaspoon finely chopped fresh thyme

freshly ground black pepper

sea salt

1 ripe tomato, thinly sliced

1 teaspoon sweet paprika

2 teaspoons dried mixed herbs

Method

1 Preheat the oven to 180°C (160°C fan-forced).

2 Grease a 25 centimetre quiche dish and line it with the pastry sheet.

3   In a bowl, combine the eggs, half the grated cheese, the cottage cheese, asparagus, capsicum, spring onion, chilli, chives, parsley, thyme, black pepper and sea salt to taste.

4   Pour the filling into the pastry-lined quiche dish and top with the remaining cheese, the tomato and a sprinkle of paprika and dried mixed herbs.

5   Bake for 20–30 minutes or until the filling is nicely browned and the pastry is well cooked.

Notes

- Serve with lots of fresh Italian-dressed salad and a tall glass of mineral water with freshly squeezed lemon juice, slices of fresh lemon and ice.
- Substitute mushrooms for asparagus for a different spin on the same recipe.
- This quiche makes a tasty, healthy lunch and is great for entertaining.
- Can be eaten cold.

Toddler tip
- Allow to cool slightly and cut into bite-sized pieces. Serve it with a mini salad cheese cubes, tomato chunks, sliced cucumber and avocado.

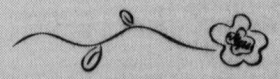

BOLOGNESE WITH PASTA

Serves 4

Ingredients

2 teaspoons extra virgin olive oil

1 large onion, finely chopped

3 garlic cloves, finely chopped

450 grams low-fat quality beef mince or vegetarian
   casserole mince, ready to use

1 large or 2 small zucchini, finely chopped

1 carrot, finely chopped

1 red capsicum, finely chopped

2 celery stalks, finely chopped

½ cup finely chopped green beans

2 tablespoons commercial gravy powder

1 cup chopped fresh tomatoes (deseeded) or 400 gram
   can diced tomatoes

1½ cups tomato pasta sauce, bought or homemade

¼ cup tomato paste

¼ teaspoon dried thyme

¼ teaspoon chilli powder (optional)

sea salt

freshly ground black pepper

500 grams whole grain pasta (spaghetti or fettuccini)

2 cups finely chopped baby spinach leaves or silverbeet, loosely packed

½ cup low-fat cheese, finely grated

1 tablespoon finely chopped fresh parsley

1 cup water

Method

1 Heat the olive oil in a deep heavy-based frying pan and cook the onion and garlic over medium heat.

2 Add the mince and cook until golden brown.

3 Add all the vegetables except the tomatoes and stir for 1–2 minutes.

4 Sprinkle the gravy powder over the mince mixture and stir it in.

5 Add the tomatoes into the pan and stir well before adding the pasta sauce, tomato paste, thyme and chilli. Season to taste with sea salt and freshly ground black pepper.

6 Add the water and bring the mince mixture to the boil, reduce the heat and allow to simmer slowly over a low heat for 20–30 minutes or until the liquid is reduced and the sauce has thickened.

7 Meanwhile, cook the pasta as directed on the packet, drain well and set aside.

8 Just before serving, stir the finely shredded baby spinach leaves into the mince mixture.

9 Arrange the pasta in individual pasta bowls and top with the mince mixture. Garnish with a sprinkle of low-fat cheese, parsley and some freshly ground black pepper.

10 Serve immediately.

Notes

- This sauce can also be used in lasagne.
- Include this sauce in a tasty pie. Place a sheet of low-fat whole grain pastry in a greased 25 centimetre

pie dish, add the sauce, then a layer of mashed sweet potato and top with another sheet of pastry. Bake in a medium oven for 45 minutes or until the pastry is golden brown. Serve with freshly steamed vegetables.

- Bulk up the fibre content in this dish by adding more vegetables.

Toddler tips

- Ensure all the vegetables are very finely chopped or grated and even the fussiest eater won't know they are eating them.

- Freeze small individual portions for easy, delicious, healthy dinners that children will love. All you'll have to do is cook some noodles and heat the sauce.

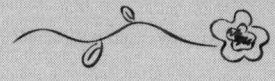

HEARTY STOCKPOT
Serves 4

Ingredients
1 tablespoon extra virgin olive oil
1 large onion, diced
2 garlic cloves, finely chopped
400 gram can vegetarian nutmeat or 400 grams gravy
    beef, cut into 1 centimetre cubes
2 tablespoons commercial gravy powder
¼ teaspoon paprika
sea salt (to taste)
freshly ground black pepper
1 teaspoon chilli (optional)
1 cup water (as needed)
1 medium zucchini, cubed
½ cup diced red capsicum
1 tablespoon sesame seeds
1 tablespoon soy sauce
3 medium sweet potatoes, cubed and partially
    cooked
1 cup pumpkin, cubed and partially cooked
2 cups cooked brown rice

Method
1 Heat the olive oil in a large heavy-based saucepan,
   add onion and garlic and cook over medium heat
   until the onion is translucent.
2 Add the nutmeat or meat and fry until it is golden
   brown.
3 Sprinkle in the gravy powder, paprika, sea salt and

freshly ground black pepper and chilli to taste, and stir well for 2 minutes, taking care not to let the mixture stick or burn.

4 Turn the temperature to high, then add the water and stir. Add the zucchini and capsicum, stirring occasionally for 3–4 minutes until the mixture comes to the boil.

5 Add the sesame seeds and soy sauce and stir for a further minute.

6 Add the pumpkin and sweet potato, reduce to low heat, stir, then cover and simmer until all the vegetables are just cooked. Add more water if needed.

7 Add the rice to the mixture and heat through.

8 Serve immediately.

Notes

- This mixture can be served on a bed of brown rice instead of mixing the rice through it.
- Top with a small dollop of extra light sour cream or natural yogurt for added richness.
- Best served hot with fresh wholemeal bread rolls, warmed slightly in the oven, and lots of fresh leafy green salad.

Toddler tips

- Omit the chilli if cooking this dish for young children.
- Mash coarsely before serving to toddlers.
- Serve with a chunk of wholemeal bread or a wholemeal roll.

BEAUT FOR THE BARBECUE BURGERS
Serves 4

Ingredients
1 tablespoon extra virgin olive oil

1 onion, chopped

2 garlic cloves, finely chopped

1 cup brown lentils, cooked or canned

1 free range egg

1 medium sweet potato, cubed and partially cooked

½ cup mashed cooked pumpkin

¼ cup peas (fresh, frozen or tinned)

½ cup finely grated zucchini

1 tablespoon soy sauce

1 tablespoon sweet chilli sauce

1 tablespoon wholemeal flour

1 tablespoon wheat germ

1 teaspoon paprika

freshly ground black pepper

sea salt

¼ cup sesame seeds

¼ cup extra wholemeal flour for coating patties

Method
1 Heat some of the olive oil in a small frying pan and partially cook the onion. Add the garlic and cook for 2–3 minutes or until the onion is translucent. Transfer the onions and garlic into a large bowl.

2 Add all the other ingredients except the sesame seeds and the ¼ cup of flour, seasoning to taste with the sea salt and black pepper.

3   In a separate bowl combine the sesame seeds with the coating flour. Set aside.

4   Create patties by taking a small amount (about the size of a small plum) and rolling it in your hands to make a ball. Roll the ball in the flour–sesame mix and flatten slightly between your hands before placing it on a lightly floured plate. Continue until the entire mixture has been used.

5   Seal the plate of patties with plastic wrap and store them in the fridge for up to 24 hours.

6   Cook on a well-oiled barbecue or in a lightly oiled non-stick frying pan, taking care to keep the patties from sticking. Flatten with a spatula to ensure that they are cooked right through, and cook on both sides until the patties are golden brown.

Notes

- Perfect for healthy burgers. Serve on unbuttered wholemeal pita bread or fat-free Turkish bread with lots of fresh salad greens, grated beetroot, grated carrot, slices of tomato, sliced onion, avocado, cucumber and sweet chilli or tomato sauce. You can spread the bread with low-fat hummus for added texture and flavour.

- For extra fibre add some ground nuts (or LSA), some roughly mashed beans or chickpeas, and increase the amount of wheat germ.

- Give the patties a Mexican flavour by adding 1 cup of red kidney beans when you fry the onions as well as some Mexican-style seasoning.

- These are delicious served as a main meal with lots of fresh green salad and a serve of sweet potato salad or tuna salad.

Toddler tips

- Make mini toddler-sized patties, leaving out the chilli, salt and black pepper.

- Serve as they are with a toddler-style salad of tomato chunks, avocado, cheese cubes, pineapple pieces, snowpeas and finely grated carrot or carrot sticks.

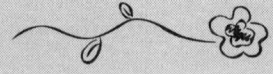

SPICY TOFU STIR FRY
Serves 4

Ingredients
2 tablespoons soy sauce
1 tablespoon honey
2 tablespoons red wine
1 teaspoon fresh red chilli, finely chopped
2 garlic cloves, finely chopped
1 centimetre piece ginger, finely grated
1 tablespoon extra virgin olive oil
1 red onion, chopped
250 grams marinated tofu
½ cup julienned carrot
½ cup julienned zucchini
½ cup julienned celery
1 cup broccoli florets
1 cup julienned red capsicum
3 spring onions, finely sliced
½ cup snowpeas, cut into strips
1 bunch bok choy or similar leafy green Asian
   vegetable
1 cup baby spinach leaves, loosely packed
1 cup bean sprouts, loosely packed
500 gram packet fresh fat-free Chinese noodles

Method
1 In a small bowl combine the soy sauce, honey,
   red wine, chilli, garlic and ginger and mix well. Set
   aside.

2 Heat the olive oil in a deep heavy-based frying pan or wok and lightly fry the onion.

3 Turn the heat to high and add the tofu, cooking until golden and crispy. Add a small amount of the prepared sauce while the tofu is cooking.

4 Add the carrot, zucchini, celery, broccoli and capsicum and fry for a further 2–3 minutes.

5 Add the spring onions, snowpeas and bok choy and cooking for 1–2 minutes before adding the spinach, bean sprouts and the prepared sauce. Turn off the heat.

6 Meanwhile, prepare the noodles as directed on the packet.

7 Toss the tofu and vegetables with the noodles, heating them through but taking care not to overcook the vegetables.

8 Serve immediately.

Notes

- This is a wonderfully quick, easy, super-healthy meal. Substitute whatever vegetables are in season, or growing in your garden that are suitable for stir-fries.

Toddler tips
- You can lightly flavour a toddler's serving as a separate batch with a simple sauce of honey and a dash of salt-reduced soy sauce.
- Cut the vegetables and the noodles into toddler-sized pieces.

Main meals

ZANY ZUCCHINI PIE
Serves 4

Ingredients
6 free range eggs, lightly beaten
1½ cups finely grated low-fat cheese
1 teaspoon finely chopped fresh parsley
1 teaspoon finely chopped fresh basil
1 tablespoon wheat germ
2 garlic cloves, finely chopped
1 teaspoon fresh red chilli, finely chopped (optional)
sea salt
freshly ground black pepper
1 cup canned whole tomatoes with herbs, drained and
    crushed
5 medium zucchinis thinly grated, with approximately
    ¼ cup sliced into thin rings
3 slices cooked bacon or vegetarian soy rashers, dried
    on paper towel and thinly sliced (optional)
1 brown onion, finely diced
1 teaspoon finely chopped fresh thyme

Method
1 Preheat the oven to 180°C (160°C fan-forced) and
   grease a rectangular baking dish.
2 Combine the eggs, 1 cup of the cheese, the parsley,
   basil, wheat germ, garlic, chilli, and sea salt and
   black pepper to taste.
3 Add the crushed tomatoes and mix gently until just
   combined.

4 Stir in the zucchini, bacon and onion.
5 Pour the mixture into the baking dish and sprinkle with the remaining cheese and the thyme.
6 Bake for 20–30 minutes or until the 'pie' is golden brown on top and firm all the way through.

Notes

- Serve this in slices with lots of hot steamed vegetables and mashed pumpkin with freshly ground black pepper and sea salt.
- Also very tasty cold as picnic food or in a packed lunch.
- Add 1 cup of grated potato and some finely chopped sun dried tomato (not in oil) for a different flavour.

Toddler tip

- Try making a separate smaller zucchini pie for toddlers, with an increased amount of cheese and no salt, pepper or chilli.

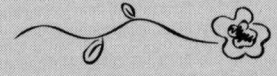

PERFECTLY PIZZA
Serves 2–4

Ingredients
1 large round wholemeal Lebanese or lavash bread
½ cup tomato paste
¼ cup thinly sliced mushrooms
1 cup finely chopped onion
3 garlic cloves, finely chopped
¼ cup fresh or canned pineapple pieces
½ cup finely chopped capsicum
2 tablespoons chopped Kalamata olives
2 ripe tomatoes, thinly sliced
2 vegetarian soy rashers or 2 slices fat-free ham, thinly
    sliced
½ cup shredded baby spinach leaves
¼ cup finely chopped spring onions
½ cup finely grated low-fat cheese
1 teaspoon mixed dried herbs
1 teaspoon finely chopped fresh thyme

Method
1 Preheat the oven to 220°C (200°C fan-forced).
2 Place the pizza base on round metal tray and layer
    on the toppings, starting with the tomato paste and
    finishing with the cheese and a sprinkle of dried
    herbs and thyme.
3 Cook in a very hot oven for 15 minutes or until
    well cooked and crispy.

Notes

- Use as many vegetables as possible on the pizza and limit the meat and olives.
- Limit a portion to half a pizza or less and serve with lots of fresh salad greens.
- For something different use skinless chicken breast or seafood, like prawns and scallops.

Toddler tip

- Make your toddler their very own pizza with extra cheese and no onions or chilli. Remove it from the oven before it becomes too crispy, and cut it into small wedges so it's easier for little ones to eat. Serve at room temperature.

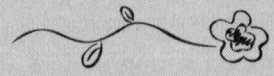

OVEN BAKED FISH WITH CRISPY SWEET POTATO WEDGES AND FRESH ITALIAN-FLAVOURED SALAD

Serves 4

Ingredients

5 sweet potatoes, unpeeled, cut into long wedges
1 teaspoon balsamic vinegar
1 teaspoon finely chopped fresh red chilli (optional)
3 garlic cloves, crushed
1 teaspoon dried mixed herbs
1 tablespoon wholemeal flour
¼ teaspoon paprika
sea salt
freshly ground black pepper
1 teaspoon extra virgin olive oil
4 fresh de-boned white fish fillets
1 large onion, thin-sliced into rings
juice of 1 lemon
juice of 1 lime
3 cups fresh salad greens (including lettuce, rocket, baby spinach leaves, Asian greens, fresh sprouts, mustard greens), loosely packed
1 avocado, chopped
2 ripe tomatoes, chopped
100 grams low-fat feta cheese, chopped into small cubes
4 olives, sliced
¼ cup freshly grated fresh beetroot
¼ cup canned corn kernels
¼ cup red capsicum, thinly sliced

1 tablespoon sunflower seeds

1 tablespoon pepitas

1 teaspoon finely chopped fresh parsley

¼ cup fat-free Italian salad dressing, bought or
homemade

Method

1 Preheat the oven to 200°C (180°C fan-forced).

2 Place the sweet potato wedges into a plastic bag
with the balsamic vinegar, chilli (optional), half the
garlic, the mixed herbs, flour, paprika, sea salt and
black pepper to taste, and the olive oil. Seal the
bag closed, then shake it vigorously until all the
wedges are lightly coated, adding a little more oil
and vinegar if necessary.

3 Place the prepared wedges onto a lightly greased
or non-stick tray and bake for 20 minutes, turning
once to allow both sides to brown.

4 Cut two large pieces of alfoil the same size that you
will use to make a giant 'envelope'. Line a baking
tray with one sheet and fold 1 centimetre of the
edges upward all the way round.

5 Lie the fish fillets on the alfoil sheet and top with
thin slices of tomato, the rest of the garlic, the onion,
freshly squeezed lemon juice, freshly squeezed lime
juice, chilli (optional), sea salt and freshly ground
black pepper to taste. Cover with the other sheet
of alfoil and fold all edges of both sheets together
to form a sealed 'oven bag' enclosing the fish.

6 When the wedges are nearly finished cooking (a fork will penetrate easily), put the tray containing the fish parcel into the oven and reduce the heat to 180°C (160°C fan-forced). Bake for 7–10 minutes or until well cooked, depending on the thickness of the fillets. Leave the fish in the 'oven bag' and increase the heat for 5 minutes or until the wedges become really crisp. Remove the fish and the wedges from the oven.

7 Meanwhile, in a large bowl, roughly shred the salad greens and add the avocado, tomato, feta cheese, olives, beetroot, corn kernels, capsicum, seeds, onion and parsley and toss together lightly.

8 Add the dressing to salad and toss through.

9 Serve one fillet of fish per plate with plenty of fresh salad and a small serve of wedges.

Notes

- Wedges can be topped with a small dollop of extra light sour cream and some sweet chilli sauce.
- This salad is an excellent filler, so serve more of it than anything else and always eat the salad first.
- Fish can be bought fresh or frozen, or caught by yourself. If buying, always look for certified sustainably-caught fish.

Toddler tip
- Chop wedges into bite-sized pieces and serve with cooked fish, cubes of cheese, tomato, avocado and some corn kernels.

SWISH VEGETABLE KEBABS WITH FLAVOURED WILD RICE

Serves 4

Ingredients

1 tablespoon soy sauce
1 tablespoon honey
1 tablespoon freshly squeezed lime juice
sea salt
freshly ground black pepper
¼ teaspoon chilli (optional)
½ teaspoon mixed dried herbs
2 chicken-flavoured stock cubes
2 garlic cloves, crushed
¼ teaspoon cumin
¼ teaspoon paprika
¼ teaspoon finely chopped fresh curly parsley
¼ teaspoon dehydrated onion
2 cups uncooked wild rice
2 red capsicums, cut into bite-sized pieces
½ fresh pineapple, peeled and cut into bite-sized pieces
1 medium eggplant, cut into bite-sized pieces
3 zucchini, cut into bite-sized pieces
250 grams skinless cooked chicken pieces, cut into bite-sized pieces (optional)
6 spring onions, finely chopped

Method

1 In a long, shallow rectangular dish combine the soy

sauce, honey, lime juice, chilli, ¼ teaspoon mixed dried herbs, and sea salt and black pepper to taste. Set aside.

2 Bring a saucepan of water to the boil (check the rice packet for the amount of water required).

3 To the boiling water add the stock cubes, 1 clove of crushed garlic, the cumin, paprika, parsley, dehydrated onion, ¼ teaspoon mixed dried herbs, and sea salt and black pepper to taste.

4 Add the rice, reduce the heat slightly and cook uncovered for the length of time prescribed on the rice packet.

5 Line a griller rack with alfoil or grease a barbecue hotplate.

6 Thread pieces of capsicum, pineapple, eggplant, zucchini and chicken onto skewers and roll them lightly in the marinade, then cook under the grill or on the barbecue until browned on all sides.

7 Drain the cooked rice, serve it in a bowl shape on individual plates, then sprinkle it with finely chopped spring onions and black pepper. Top with the kebab sticks and drizzle with a little extra marinade.

8 Serve immediately.

Notes

- Substitute marinated tofu for the chicken if you want a vegetarian version.
- Serve two kebabs with some fresh salad greens as a delicious healthy lunch for one.

Toddler tip

- Remove the food from the sticks before serving to toddlers or very young children.

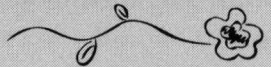

TASTY TUNA RICE
Serves 4

Ingredients
1 tablespoon extra virgin olive oil
1 onion, diced
2 garlic cloves, finely chopped
¼ teaspoon paprika
sea salt
freshly ground black pepper
3 zucchinis, chopped into small pieces
¼ cup spring onion, finely chopped
1 large red capsicum, chopped into small pieces
400 gram can tuna in spring water, drained
juice of ½ a lemon
2 tablespoons kecap-manis thick sweet soy sauce
¼ cup fresh green beans, chopped into small pieces
½ cup canned corn kernels
¼ cup fresh snowpeas, chopped into small pieces
3 cups cooked and drained brown rice
1 teaspoon finely chopped fresh parsley

Method
1 Heat the olive oil in a heavy-based frying pan and sauté the onion and garlic.
2 Add the paprika and sea salt and black pepper to taste. Stir through.
3 Add the zucchini, spring onion and capsicum and cook for a further 2–3 minutes.
4 Add the tuna and mix it through, then add the

lemon juice, soy sauce and green beans, stirring for 2–3 minutes.

5   Mix through all the remaining ingredients including the drained rice, except the parsley, and season with sea salt and black pepper to taste.

6   Serve topped with some finely chopped parsley and spring onions.

Notes

- Yellow zucchini can be used for a more colourful presentation.
- Organic cooked chick peas are a great addition to this dish.
- Finely chopped fresh red chilli can be added for some extra heat.
- You can use tasty tuna rice to stuff capsicums, baked potatoes or large squash.
- Try serving as a side dish with a piece of grilled skinless chicken or fish.
- Leave the tuna out for a vegetarian version.

Toddler tip

- During the cooking process set aside a small portion for the little ones before seasoning with salt, to reduce the salt content of their serving.

- Serve to toddlers with some mashed potato.

BEAN TACOS
Serves 4

Ingredients
4 cups of soft lettuce leaves, loosely packed
1 cup finely grated carrot
3 ripe tomatoes, diced
1 cup finely grated fresh beetroot
2 cups finely grated low-fat cheese
1 cup finely chopped spring onion
1 cup thinly sliced capsicum
2 ripe avocados, thinly sliced
1 teaspoon extra virgin olive oil
1 onion, chopped
435 gram can refried beans
420 gram can baked beans or 420 gram can red kidney
    beans, washed and drained
1 packet taco seasoning mix
¼ teaspoon finely chopped fresh red chilli
    (optional)
½ cup water
12 large taco shells

Method
1 Preheat the oven to 180°C (160°C fan-forced).
2 Assemble the lettuce, carrot, tomato, beetroot, cheese, spring onion, capsicum and avocado either in individual bowls or on a platter.
3 Heat the olive oil in a heavy-based saucepan and cook the onion until it is transparent.

4 Add the refried beans and baked beans, stir into the onion, then add the taco seasoning mix, chilli and water, mixing together well.

5 Simmer uncovered over medium heat, stirring until the liquid has reduced, then lower the heat and roughly mash the beans while they are still in the saucepan.

6 Heat the taco shells in the oven for 1 minute or until warm to the touch.

7 Spoon the bean mixture into a large shallow bowl in the centre of the table alongside the salad ingredients and taco shells. Invite everyone to assemble their own tacos.

Notes

- To reduce individual serve sizes this can be served with a dressed side salad.
- Either baked beans or red kidney beans can be used. Baked beans give a sweeter flavour because they contain added sugar, but red kidney beans are a healthier option.
- A small dollop of extra light sour cream can be added on top of each taco.
- You can serve pre-assembled tacos to reduce mess and ensure that everyone has plenty of salad in their tacos.

Toddler tips

- Don't overload the tacos or they will be difficult for little ones to eat.

- Serve some of the bean mix in a bowl with a spoon, alongside another bowl containing chopped tomato, cubes of cheese, cubes of cucumber, slices of avocado and grated carrot and fresh beetroot.

- Try making a toasted sandwich for the little ones with whole grain bread, the bean mixture and cheese. Serve with their own little salad of cubes of tomato, slices of avocado and some finely grated carrot and fresh beetroot.

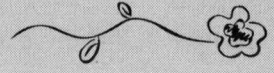

SPROUT STIR FRY
Serves 4

Ingredients
1 tablespoon extra virgin olive oil
1 onion, chopped
1½ cups cubed vegetarian nutmeat
2 garlic cloves, finely chopped
1 centimetre piece ginger, peeled and finely chopped
1 teaspoon finely chopped fresh red chilli (optional)
1 tablespoon soy sauce
1 teaspoon sesame seeds
1 tablespoon freshly squeezed lemon juice
125 grams mushrooms, sliced
3 slices fat-free ham (optional)
1 bunch bok choy, rinsed, drained and chopped
1 cup large bean sprouts
1 cup baby spinach leaves, loosely packed

Method
1 Heat the olive oil in a large heavy-based frying pan or a wok.
2 Add onion to the hot oil, fry for 3 minutes or until slightly transparent, then add the nutmeat and fry until golden brown.
3 Add the garlic, ginger, chilli, soy sauce, sesame seeds and lemon juice. Allow them to form a kind of paste, then stir through.
4 Add the mushrooms and ham and stir for 1–2 minutes.

5   Add the bok choy and sprouts and stir for a further
    minute until they wilt. Add the spinach and quickly
    toss it through before turning off the heat.
6   Serve immediately.

Notes
- Serve with wholegrain toast.
- Add some extra light sour cream at the end to make
  a creamier sauce.
- For a non-vegetarian version substitute thin strips
  of cooked lean beef or chicken for the nutmeat.
- Use vegetables in season for really fresh results.
- Perfect for serving to vegetarian guests if you leave
  out the ham.

Toddler tip
- Serve toddlers a portion with some noodles, raw
  snowpeas, carrot sticks and pieces of cooked
  chicken, nutmeat or strips of beef.

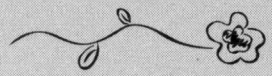

Acknowledgements

I would like to thank the following people who have helped me to bring this book to you:

My beautiful daughter Lily, you are such a light in my life. You are my inspiration. Damien, my fiancé, I love you so much. My mother, who has always been so supportive and loving and brought me up to always embrace my creative side. My Aunty Shirley, who is such an amazing, intelligent and talented woman. My step-mother, Colleen, who is so talented, caring and accomplished. My grandmother who has passed away, and my grandfather, I love you so much. My dad, you are such a great man. I only need to think of you and I smile. My family and my extended family, I love you all. Shirlene Harris, thank you for so much during my childhood.

Sophie Hamley, my wonderful and fabulous agent, thank you so very much for everything and making this all happen. Roberta Ivers, my editor, you are a sensational woman, you have taken such care of me and this book, I cannot thank you enough. Nikki Christer, Katie Stackhouse and Jill Brown for believing in my book and making it happen. The rest of the talented team at Random House who have worked with my book, in particular Annabel Rijks, my publicist, and the fantastic sales and marketing departments, you are such a wonderful group of people, thanks so much. And to Desney Shoemark, you are truly gifted!

Cherie Curtis, thank you for all your support and advice. Cristel Simmonds and the fabulous team at the *Bundaberg News Mail*, thanks for all your wonderful support. Lisa Blainey-Lewin, you are such an encouraging and inspirational woman, your energy and enthusiasm is infectious, thank you from the bottom of my heart. Thanks too, to Debra Murphy, Joan Dooley, Margaret Wass and Shani Jamieson; and also to Kat and Paul Poco from the mothering site bellyhood.com. Irene Bates, who gave me such guidance and encouragement during my time at Bunnings, you are a real jewel. Thanks to Bill Webb, Manager of Bunnings in Bundaberg, and also Joy, Desley, Anna, Kylie, Sheena, Sorelle, Julie, Grant, Kelly, Nola and the rest of the great team I worked with there.

Ange and Jarad, you, too, have been such a big part of our lives, we love you. Fiona, Susan and Jodie,

thank you for appearing on television with me
Pirkko and all my friends, thank you.

All the wonderful women and mothers I know,
and those I have met and who have supported me
through my page on MySpace and this book, you are
fantastic!

Rebecca Mugridge